Acoustic Emission: Probes and Utilization

Contents

Preface

A variety of information related to acoustic emission has been compiled in this book. Acoustic Emission (AE) is a phenomenon in which elastic or stress waves are produced from speedy, localized change of strain energy in substances. The practical function of AE first emerged in the 1950s, but it is only in the last two decades that the science, technology and applications of AE have progressed notably. At present, AE has become one of the most significant non-destructive testing methods. This multidisciplinary book contains data which demonstrates that the AE method is constantly rising and extensively functional in on-line monitoring of civil-engineering constructions such as flyovers, buildings, etc. AE is also applied for the exposure of fatigue cracks and their positions in complex vessels and pipelines, damage estimation in fiber-toughened polymer-matrix compounds, among others. This book will be helpful for both students and experts interested in this field.

This book has been the outcome of endless efforts put in by authors and researchers on various issues and topics within the field. The book is a comprehensive collection of significant researches that are addressed in a variety of chapters. It will surely enhance the knowledge of the field among readers across the globe.

It is indeed an immense pleasure to thank our researchers and authors for their efforts to submit their piece of writing before the deadlines. Finally in the end, I would like to thank my family and colleagues who have been a great source of inspiration and support.

Editor

Hit Detection and Determination in AE Bursts

Rúnar Unnþórsson

Additional information is available at the end of the chapter

1. Introduction

This chapter presents a methodology for detecting and determining Acoustic Emission (AE) hits in AE bursts, i.e. signals with large number of overlapping transients with variable strengths. The methodology is designed to overcome important limitations of threshold-based approaches in determining hits in this type of AE signal; for example, when the signal's amplitude between transients does not fall below the threshold for a predetermined period of time. The threshold-based approach is a special case of the proposed methodology. The methodology, and the associated algorithms, were presented in *Acoustic Emission-Based Fatigue Failure Criterion for CFRP* by Runar Unnthorsson, Thomas P. Runarsson and Magnus T. Jonsson [17] and used in four articles by the same authors [15, 16, 18, 19].

The chapter is organized as follows. Section 2 provides the reader with an overview of Acoustic Emissions, what they are, how they are acquired and the various factors that can affect them from when they are emitted until they are digitized by the AE system. Majority of these factors will change the originally emitted AE waves so that the digitized representation will be different. In Section 3 an overview of the AE processing techniques is given with emphasis on conventional methods of determining AE hits and the corresponding hit parameters. The section also introduces the problem of determining AE hits in bursts. Section 4 then introduces the methodology and presents the algorithms. In section 5 an experimental AE signal is used to demonstrate the methodology. The chapter ends with section 6 which concludes the chapter and provides suggestions for future research into this topic.

2. Acoustic Emissions

Acoustic Emission (AE) is a term used for transient elastic stress waves generated by the energy released when microstructural changes occur in a material [9, 21]. The energy is provided by an elastic stress field in the material. The stress field can be generated by stressing the material, for instance using mechanical, thermal, pressure and chemical stressing. These types of stress all contribute to fatigue failure and are commonly encountered in-service. As the stress waves propagate from the AE source they are influenced by a variety of factors. These factors include propagation velocities, attenuation, reflection, refraction, discontinuities and the geometry of the material. Furthermore, the propagation velocity of an elastic stress wave depends on the wave type, material properties and frequency. When the stress waves reach the surface they cause it to vibrate and the vibration can be measured. The minute surface displacements are measured using sensitive transducers which respond to surface displacements to the order of several picometers. Several types of transducers can be used for this: piezoelectric, capacitance, electromagnetic and optical. The last two are non-contact, but electromagnetic transducers are considerably less sensitive than piezoelectric transducers. Optical sensors, e.g. laser, are free of resonance and can be absolutely calibrated by measuring the correct amplitude of the AE [8].

Piezoelectric transducers are the most popular and are either of a broadband or a resonance type. The transducers are made by using a special ceramic, usually Porous Lead Zirconate Titanate (PZT). Figure 1 shows a schematic view of a piezoelectric transducer and how an AE is converted into an electric representation. The transducers are pressed up against the surface of the material and the vibration is transferred to the PZT inside the transducer through the wear plate. When the PZT element vibrates it generates an electric signal. The transducer's signal is, therefore, a 1D voltage-time representation of the 3D displacement-time wave that it senses.

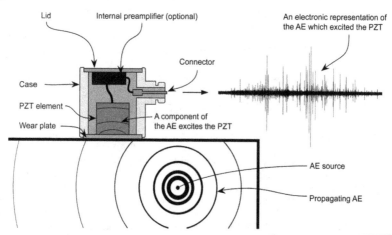

Figure 1. An illustration of a typical resonant piezoelectric AE transducer and how an AE is converted into an electric representation.

Measurements using piezoelectric transducers are sensitive to how the vibration is transferred to them. The main factors that affect this are: the material's surface, the transducer's pressure against the material, and the coupling medium [5]. The presence of a transducer affects the vibration; however, this is unavoidable when using contact transducers. The direction of the waves also affect the transducer's response. This is because AE transducers are nearly always designed to measure the components of the AE waves that are normal to the surface [1]. Although the stress waves typically have components in the normal direction this directionality means that the response to identical waves arriving from different directions will not be the same.

The selection of transducers is most often based on their frequency response curves, also known as calibration curves. These curves can be absolute or relative. The most typical calibration curves are relative displacement and pressure response curves. Relative curves are useful for comparison of transducers. At Vallen Systeme GmbH pressure and displacement curves are generated by connecting an exciter face to face with the corresponding transducer [20]. In both cases continuous sine waves are used for excitation. Pressure curves are generated by exciting the sensing area uniformly, but displacement curves are performed by using an exciter with small aperture size. The displacement calibration is an attempt to simulate line excitation of a travelling displacement wave. Figure 2 demonstrates the difference between these two calibration methods. The red curve is the result of a pressure calibration and the green curve is the result of a displacement calibration. The resulting response curves are more relevant for continuous and long duration AE signals than for transient AE signals. Some authors have deconvolved the AE signal with the frequency response of the transducers as an attempt to minimize the effect of the rugged frequency response of resonant transducers [7, 11]. The transducer's response to transient signals is, however, different from the response to continuous waves. Hence, the convolution may not work as intended or even make things worse.

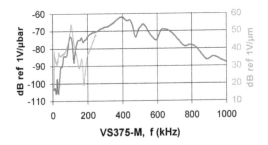

Figure 2. Two calibration curves for the same resonant AE transducer. The red curve is the result of a pressure calibration and the green is the result of a displacement calibration (reproduced with permission from Vallen GmbH).

3. Conventional AE processing and hit detection

Due to all the influencing factors listed above, the digitized representation of the AE will be different from the original emission. Despite this, and somewhat surprising, acquired AEs have been successfully used to detect, monitor and distinguish between several damages, e.g. delamination, matrix cracking, debonding, fibre cracking and fibre pull-outs in fibre-reinforced polymer composites [3, 4, 10, 12, 21, 22].

Acoustic Emission signals can be roughly divided into three types: bursts, continuous and mixed [6]. Bursts are transient signals generated by the formation of damage, e.g. fiber breaking and delamination. Continuous AE signals are generated when multiple transients overlap so that they cannot be distinguished and the envelope of the signal amplitudes becomes constant. Continuous AE can be generated by electrical noise and rubbing. The mixed type signal contains both bursts and continuous signals and it is the type which is normally encountered in-service.

Over the years many research projects have been conducted with the aim of extracting useful information from AE signals. The extracted information is stored in n-dimensional data structures, known as features. A number of techniques can be used for extracting the AE features. A popular method is to identify transient waves in the signal and extract the features from them. These transients, also called hits, are therefore portions of the measured AE waveform which satisfy a given detection criterion. The purpose of the detection criterion is to detect the presence of transient AE and discriminate it from background noise, or continuous AE. Because AE are mainly transient stress waves, the term AE hit is usually understood as an isolated, and separated, transient from the acquired waveform.

There are many detection techniques which can be used for detecting and determining AE hits. A common technique used in realtime commercial parameter-based AE systems is to compare the AE signal against a certain threshold. The threshold is typically set on the positive side of the signal, just above the noise, and held fixed. The threshold is sometimes floating, i.e. it is adjusted regularly so that it is just above the noise. A hit is detected by comparing the AE signal against the threshold and if the signal surpasses the threshold a hit is detected. Figure 3 illustrates the threshold based hit detection and shows how few well established features are computed.

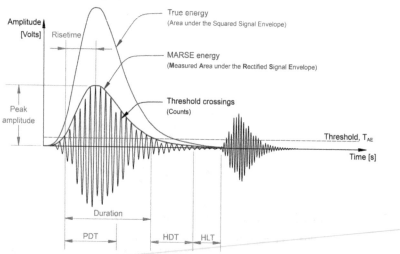

Figure 3. Illustration of the threshold based hit detection and the AE features extracted from each hit.

After an AE hit has been detected it is determined. Three parameters are commonly used with the determination of AE hits: the hit definition time (HDT), the hit lockout time (HLT), and the peak definition time (PDT). These parameters are illustrated in Fig. 3. The HDT parameter specifies the maximum time between threshold crossing, i.e. if no crossing occurs during this time then the hit has ended. If the HDT is set too high then the system may consider two or more hits as one. If the HDT is set too low then the system may not fully capture the AE hit and possibly treat one hit as multiple ones. The HLT parameter specifies time which must pass after an hit has been detected before a new hit can be detected. If the HLT is set too high then the system may not capture the next AE and if it is set too low then the system may capture reflections and late arriving component of the AE as hits. The PDT parameter specifies the time allowed, after a hit has been detected, to determine the peak value. If the PDT is set too high then false measurements of peak value are more likely to occur. It is recommended that the PDT should be set as low as possible. However care must be taken not to set it too low because that may result in the true peak not being identified.

Once the AE hit has been determined hit-based features can be extracted. Conventional AE hit-based features include amplitude, duration, energy, number of peaks above certain threshold (ring-down count) and rise time [2]. Figure 3 illustrates how these and other common hit based features are related. New features can be designed by processing existing ones. The processing includes, but is not limited to: adding, subtracting, multiplying, and dividing two or more features. New features can also be made by filtering and extracting statistical information from the features in the set; e.g., variance, skewness and kurtosis.

Trend analysis of hit-based features is widely used. Sometimes trending is carried out by plotting the cumulative sum of the feature. In some applications trending can be sufficient; e.g. when monitoring of the AE signal's power alone is of interest. In many cases, however, further analysis is required. In some cases more information about a feature can be gleaned by studying its statistical parameters and its correlation with other features.

The threshold based hit technique is suitable when the background noise level is either constant or changes gradually. The threshold level is then set at the beginning of monitoring and if a floating threshold is used then the threshold is updated regularly. The technique, however, does not perform well when the AE signal contains strong temporal bursts of high AE activity. Such bursts consist of overlapping transients with varying strength, duration, shape and frequency. For this reason, the burst threshold based technique cannot determine the exact start and end of individual hits as the AE burst never drops below the threshold. Bursts with these properties occur in CFRP assemblies subjected to dynamic loading; e.g., the CFRP prosthetic foot Variflex [14, 17].

Figures 4 and 5 show the AE acquired at two different times while the Variflex was subjected to multi-axial cyclic loading. Figure 4 shows the measured AE signal during one loading cycle early during testing. Also shown, is the threshold which was set just above the noise.

Figure 5 shows the AE signal few thousand loading cycles later. The two strong bursts contain AE from many sources such as damage growth, rubbing of crack surfaces and friction between the fibres and the matrix due to their different material properties. As can be observed, the threshold based approach is not able to separate the transients in the bursts. In the next section a technique designed to overcome the abovementioned limitations of the threshold based hit detection.

4. A new methodology for detecting and determining AE hits

Transients in AE signals acquired from complex systems are often difficult or even impossible to separate using a conventional threshold based approach. There can be several reasons for this such as variable amplitude of the continuous AE within a loading cycle and overlapping of transients, which can be simultaneously emitted from the many AE sources in the material;

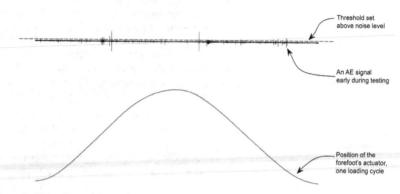

Figure 4. AE signal in one fatique cycle early during cyclic testing of an assembled CFRP.

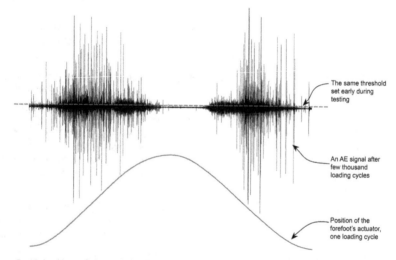

Figure 5. AE signal in one fatique cycle few thousand cycles into the cyclic test of an assembled CFRP.

e.g. in CRFP composites subjected to dynamic loading. These transients have varying strength, duration, shape, and frequency. Hence, as the complexity of the AE signal increases, more advanced signal processing methods are required to detect and separate transients.

In this section a new methodology for detecting and determining AE hits is introduced and explained. Figure 6 shows a flow chart of the procedure. In the first step, the acquired AE signal is processed in order to extract descriptive features for detection. The resulting signal is called a detection function, or novelty function, and can be in any suitable domain of interest; e.g., time and time-scale/time-frequency domains. For detecting and locating hits, the detection function is input to a peak-picking algorithm which automatically detects hits based on the trough-to-peak difference of local troughs and peaks. In the final step, the detected transients are compared against a threshold both to locate the hits more accurately, as well as to filter out weak hits; e.g., from background noise.

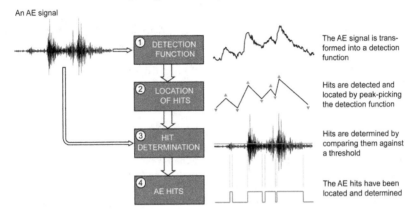

Figure 6. Flow chart of the AE hit determination procedure.

4.1. Detection functions

Two detection functions based on the signal's power will now be introduced, one in the time domain and one in the time-frequency domain.

4.1.1. Time Domain

Assuming an acceptable signal-to-noise ratio (SNR), most transients can be detected in the time domain using the temporal characteristics of the signal; e.g., the amplitude. Temporal amplitude increase is one of the key properties of transients and is, for an example, used in threshold based hit detection and determination. The signal's power can also be used for generating a detection function. In digital signal processing it is customary to refer to the squared values of a sequence as power and to the sum as energy. Hence, the power can be calculated by squaring the amplitudes:

$$P[i] = \frac{|x[i]|^2}{R} \qquad (1)$$

where x is the voltage of the acquired AE signal, R is the equivalent resistance of the transducer and amplifiers and the use of square brackets serves as a reminder that the values are discrete. In acoustics, the energy is commonly expressed in base-10 logarithm scale, known as the decibel (dB). The logarithm transformation changes the dynamic range of the signal by enhancing low values, while compressing high values. The logarithmically converted energy can be expressed by

$$P_{\log_{10}}[i] = 10\log_{10}|P[i]| = 10\log_{10}\left|\frac{|x[i]|^2}{R}\right| = -10\log_{10}|R| + 20\log_{10}|x[i]| \qquad (2)$$

Because the hits will be determined by peak-picking the detection function, both the negative constant involving R and the multiplication by 20 can be omitted. Furthermore, in order to ensure that the detection function will be positive and to eliminate the need to deal with numbers less than one, whose logarithms are negative, the rectified signal values are incremented by one. The resulting detection function is:

$$DF[i] = \log_{10}|1 + |x[i]|| \qquad (3)$$

This detection function has the shape of the the signal's power envelope. In some instances the detection function may be too jagged to accurately perform peak-picking. In order to improve the peak-picking the detection function can be filtered but, with the cost of higher computational load and a time-lag of peaks. Figure 7 illustrates the process of generating the detection function.

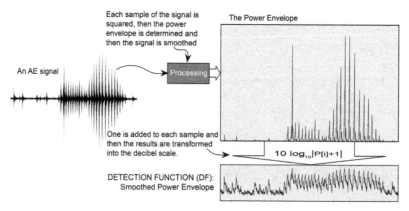

Figure 7. Illustration of the procedure for generating detection function in the time domain. In the chapter, a simplified version of this procedure is used.

4.1.2. Time-Frequency Domain

AE signals are mainly transient stress waves with a broadband frequency response. This property can also be used to detect transients. Power spectrum analysis, for instance using FFT, only shows which frequencies exist in the signal and how they are distributed. This is because the FFT is not designed to analyze transient signals, but rather continuous signals. Time-frequency representations are methods designed to analyze time-varying signals. Among the methods that have been used for this task is the Short-Time Fourier Transform (STFT).

The STFT is an enhanced version of the standard FFT. The idea behind the STFT is to divide the signal into portions where it is stationary. A window function is used to extract the portions from the original signal. The portions are then processed using FFT. Hence, the STFT is basically a FFT with a window function. The time-frequency localization obtained is from the location of the window functions. The frequency localization suffers due to the limited size of the window. For a given window size, the STFT has a constant localization resolution at all times and frequencies. By increasing the window size, the frequency localization can be improved, but then the time localization gets worse, and vice versa. This problem is related to the Heisenberg's Uncertainty Principle, which can be applied to time-frequency localization of signals. Basically what it says is that we cannot know both the exact localization of time and frequency.

In the time-frequency domain the power of the signal can also be used to detect and isolate transients. For this purpose a function based on the short-time Fourier transform can be used to generate the detection function. Figure 8 and Algorithm 1 describe how the STFT based detection function is computed.

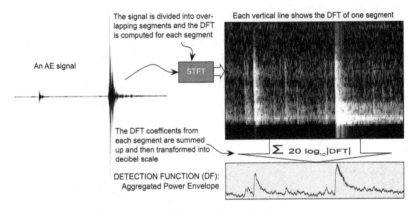

Figure 8. Illustration of how the time-frequency based detection function is generated.

The computation procedure starts by dividing the AE signal into segments of k samples. The segments overlap by d samples. For each segment, the discrete Fourier transform (DFT) is computed using k samples; i.e., no zero padding is used. Then the results are converted into the decibel scale by applying logarithm (base 10) to the complex modulus (magnitude) of the DFT coefficients. The coefficients for each segment are then summed up. Each coefficient is multiplied by a 20. The multiplication can be omitted because it only scales the detection function; i.e., the peak-picking results will be the same with adjusted parameters.

The number of elements in the detection function, DF, is equal to the number of segments. Consequently, the elements are mapped to the corresponding data points in the AE signal, the mapping is stored in a vector MAP. The time resolution is controlled by the length of the segments. The additional information obtained by using overlapping, is obtained by interpolation.

Algorithm 1: *STFT based detection function*

    Data: signal, k, d
    Result: DF, MAP

1 Segments ← signal divided into k sample segments with d sample overlap;
2 MAP ← map the segments to corresponding data points in the signal;
3 **for** *i=1* **to** number_of_segments **do**
4 | DFT ← Calculate Discrete Fourier Transform of segment *i*;
5 | DF [i] ← sum ($20\log_{10}$ (|DFT |));
6 **end**

Given the reduction in the time resolution and the computational cost involved, the STFT based detection function does not compare well against the previous detection function, which was in the time domain.

4.2. Peak-picking the detection function

In order to locate hits from the detection function a peak-picking procedure is used. The procedure is illustrated in Fig. 9. The small troughs and peaks in the detection function are incrementally removed until it contains only troughs and peaks which have trough-to-peak difference above the trough-to-peak threshold, T_{tp}. The hits are then located from the remaining troughs in the detection function. The threshold controls the sensitivity of the approach. If the sensitivity is increased; i.e., T_{tp} is lowered, then smaller pulsations in the AE signal will be detected as hits. This procedure can be split into two algorithms: Algorithm 2 and Algorithm 3.

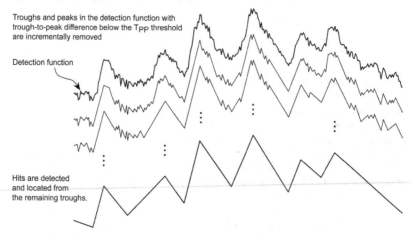

Figure 9. Illustration of the incremental peak picking procedure.

Algorithm 2 is used for locating troughs and peaks in an input signal. The algorithm starts by creating an empty vector, *Locs*, of the same length as the input signal. This vector will be the output of the algorithm and contains the locations of all detected troughs and peaks. The derivative, or slope, of the input signal is used to determine troughs and peaks. The slope is computed by subtracting a time-shifted version of the input signal from itself. Peaks are detected by first finding all samples which have zero or positive slope. If the next sample in time has negative slope then a peak is detected. The procedure for finding troughs is similar, in this case all samples with zero or negative slope are first found and when the next sample in time has positive slope then a trough is detected. The end points are treated separately. In both cases, it is first checked if a peak or trough have been determined at the ends. If not, then a trough is determined if a peak is closest to the end, and vice versa.

Algorithm 2: *Trough and Peak Picking Algorithm*

Data: signal
Result: Locs

1 Locs ← zero vector of the same size as signal;
2 *peaks:*
3 tmp_indices1 ← indices of all samples with positive slope (and 0);
4 tmp_indices2 ← indices of samples in tmp_indices1 for which the adjacent samples with indices tmp_indices1 +1 have negative slope;
5 Locs [tmp_indices1 [tmp_indices2]+1] ← (+1);
6 *valleys:*
7 tmp_indices1 ← indices of all samples with negative slope (and 0);
8 tmp_indices2 ← indices of samples in tmp_indices1 for which the adjacent samples with indices tmp_indices1 +1 have positive slope;
9 Locs [tmp_indices1 [tmp_indices2]+1] ← (-1);
10 *end points:*
11 nz_indices ← find the indices of non zero entries in Locs;
12 **if** abs (nz_indices [*first entry*]) $\neq$ 1 **then**
13 | Locs [1] ← $(-1) \times$ nz_indices [1]
14 **end**
15 **if** abs (nz_indices [*last entry*]) $\neq$ *length of signal* **then**
16 | Locs [1] ← $(-1) \times$ nz_indices [last entry]
17 **end**

Algorithm 3 is used to remove troughs and peaks which have trough-to-peak difference below a specified threshold, T_{tp}. They are removed incrementally by increasing the threshold, a, from 1 to T_{tp} in steps. The larger the increments, the larger can the hit location error be. Smaller increments, however, increase the computational cost. After each removal step, Algorithm 2 is used to reevaluate the troughs and peaks from the remaining list. The reevaluated list is then used for the next step. The hit locations determined by the peak-picking procedure are the trough locations in the final list.

4.3. Hit determination

After the hits have been located they are compared against a determination threshold, T_{AE}. This threshold is the same threshold as used in the conventional threshold-based hit detection. Here, this threshold is used to filter out weak hits; i.e., only hits which exceed the threshold are determined as hits. The threshold is also used to extract threshold based features.

Algorithm 3: *Trough and Peak Removal Algorithm*

Data: Locs, signal, T_{tp}
Result: NewLocs

1 **for** $a=1$ **to** T_{tp} **do**
2   Remove trough/peak entries in Locs which have trough-to-peak difference below a;
3   Locs_tmp ← Algorithm 2 (signal [Locs]));
4   Locs ← map the entries in Locs_tmp to entries in signal;
5 **end**
6 NewLocs ← Locs;

4.4. Summary

Continuous parameter based AE systems commonly use threshold based hit detection with a fixed or a floating threshold. However, in some situations neither may be appropriate. When the fixed threshold is set, it is tuned to the AE signal; i.e., the noise level, at the start of monitoring. As the component under monitoring degrades and the signal level increases, the threshold may not be used to detect individual transients. That is, the threshold based approach may not be able to separate transients if the signal does not fall below the threshold for a sufficient period of time. In some situations a floating threshold can be used to overcome this problem, however, a floating threshold may not be appropriate if the signal level varies. This is because it can be difficult to set the appropriate response time of the floating threshold. If it is set too fast it can be affected by strong transients.

In this section an approach for hit determination has been introduced. This approach is designed to handle the abovementioned limitations of the threshold based hit determination approaches. In order to accomplish this, hits are first detected by peak picking a detection function and then they are compared against a threshold in order to filter out weak ones. Hence, the approach is able to detect and separate transients even though the signal does not fall below the threshold. The separation is accomplished by splitting the transients at the point of lowest amplitude between them, Fig. 10 illustrates this.

5. Experimental study

In this section the approach will be studied by applying both detection functions on the same AE signal. The AE signal was obtained during cyclic testing a CFRP prosthetic foot [17]. The signal consists of 3 AE signals chosen to demonstrates the ability of the approach to work with and detect transients which amplitudes differ by magnitudes.

The AE data was sensed and amplified using the VS375-M transducer and the AEP3 preamplifier from Vallen Systeme GmbH. The preamplifier was equipped with 110 kHz high pass and 630 kHz low pass filter. The gain was set to 49 dB. The analogue AE signal was fed to a 16 bit analogue/digital (A/D) converter for a full waveform digitization using 1.25 MHz sampling rate. After digitization the data was high-pass filtered in order to remove DC and other low frequency disturbances. Phaseless filtering was used on the AE signal in order to

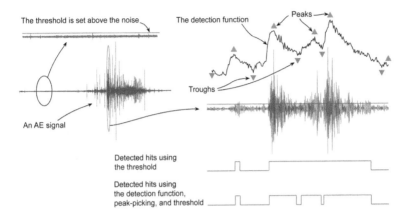

Figure 10. Illustration of how the hit determination approach presented here is able to detect and separate overlapping transients which the threshold based procedure does not.

avoid phase delay. A fifth-order elliptic filter with 1 dB passband ripple and corner frequency of 80 kHz was used. The stopband attenuation was set to 30 dB at 50 kHz. Only high pass filtering was applied to the signal. No corrections were made due to the amplifications made by the preamplifier and the transducer.

The AE signal is depicted in Fig. 11 and consists of weak, intermediate, and strong AE transients. The duration of each type is 5 milliseconds and they are arranged in the order of increasing amplitude. The weak transients are low amplitude transients, all with amplitudes equal to, or less than, 85 mV, the intermediate transients are at most 650 mV, and the strong AE transients are roughly ten times stronger, or up to 6.2 V. The strong transients have been soft clipped by the preamplifier.

In the time domain a 15 sample moving average of the power envelope was calculated before transforming it into the decibel scale. The trough-to-peak threshold, T_{tp}, was set to 13 dB V-s. The resulting detection function, which has the shape of the signal's power envelope, is plotted above the signal in Figure 12(a). The detection function has been offset to fit in the figure.

The STFT detection function described in Sect. 4.1 was used with segment size of $k = 128$ samples and $d = 120$ sample overlapping. The trough-to-peak threshold, T_{tp}, was set to 304 dB V-s. This value was used in [17] to design an AE failure criterion equivalent to a 10% displacement failure criterion. The resulting detection function is plotted above the signal in Figure 12(b)

At first sight the two detection functions may seem to be identical. However, upon close comparison one can see that they respond differently to some transients; e.g., the 3rd transient from the end of the weak transient signal portion (0-5 ms) is better defined in the time-frequency detection function. The reason for the differences lies in the nature of how the functions are generated. In the time domain the detection function is generated by squaring the signal's values, averaging them and then transforming the results into the

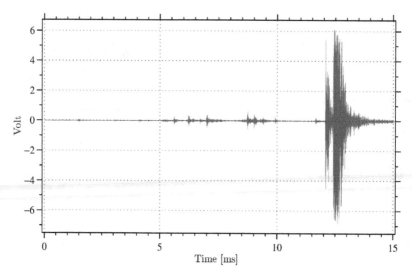

Figure 11. The AE signal that will be used to study the AE hit detection approach. The signal consists of weak (0-5 ms), intermediate (5-10 ms), and strong transients (10-15 ms).

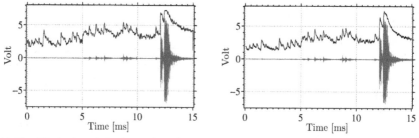

(a) The AE signal used in this study and the corresponding detection function in the time domain.

(b) The AE signal used in this study and the corresponding detection function in the time-frequency domain.

Figure 12. The two figures show the AE signal used here. The signal consists of weak, intermediate and strong transients. Above the AE signal are the two detection functions which have the shape of the signal's power envelope.

decibel scale. In the time domain, however, the frequency content of the signal is used for generating the detection function. This means that in order for an transient to have high energy both the amplitude and the frequency content play a role. Hence, the detection function in the time-frequency domain has the potential to be better at detecting the start of transients.

5.1. Weak hits

Figure 13 shows the weak transients, the two detection functions and the results from the peak-picking of the detection functions; i.e., the detected troughs and peaks. The peaks and troughs are shown respectively by triangles pointing up and down. The figure allows for better comparison of the two detection functions. In the time domain the detection function closely follows the signal's envelope whereas in the time-frequency domain the detection function does not follow the signa's envelope as well. An example is the 3rd transient from the end, located approximately at 3.8 ms. In the time domain the detection function shows the transient as a bump in the curve but, the time-domain detection function responds differently and represents it as a well defined peak. As a result, when the two detection functions are peak-picked the algorithm finds more accurate location of the peak in the time-frequency domain.

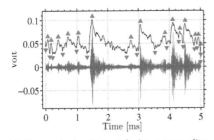
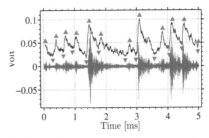

(a) The weak transients and the corresponding detection function in the time domain.

(b) The weak transients and the corresponding detection function in the time-frequency domain.

Figure 13. The figures show the weak transients, the detection functions in more detail. Also shown are the results from the peak-picking of the detection functions; i.e., the detected troughs and peaks.

More accurate location of peaks is in general obtained using the time-frequency detection function; e.g., for transients that start at 1.4 ms and 3.8 ms. However, the purpose of the peak-picking is to detect transients. The determination is performed using conventional threshold approaches. Therefore, even though the peak-picking algorithm does not provide exact timing of peaks and troughs it can be used to separate transients.

5.2. Intermediate hits

Figure 14 shows the intermediate transient. The maximum amplitude of the transient in the intermediate signal is approximately 640 mV. The amplitude is 7-8 times higher than the weak transients which are all less than one tick on the Volt axis in the figure.

It is interesting to see that, despite that the same settings are used and the transients are much stronger, the approach handles the AE signal with the intermediate transients quite well. Visual inspection and comparison of Figures 14(a) and 14(b) reveals that the peak-picking results are similar to the results when working with the weak transients.

However, inspection also shows that the detection function in the time-frequency domain can combine two or more transients into one. An example of this is the transients starting at 6.2 ms and 6.4 ms. The detection function in the time domain separates them with two peaks but in the time-frequency domain they are treated as one. This may be of the strong broadband content of the first transient which blends into the second one but, it is also due to the size of the overlapping used in the STFT calculations. The reason why the two transients are not

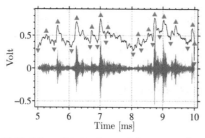

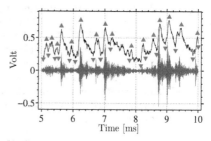

(a) The intermediate transients and the corresponding detection function in the time domain.

(b) The weak transients and the corresponding detection function in the time-frequency domain.

Figure 14. The figures show the intermediate transients, the detection functions in more detail. Also shown are the results from the peak-picking of the detection functions; i.e., the detected troughs and peaks.

identified from peak-picking the detection function in the time domain is the value of the T_{tp} - a lower value will identify the smaller transient.

5.3. Strong hits

Figure 15 shows the strong transients. The transients were soft-clipped by the amplifier but the high-pass filtering of the signal partly restored them. The maximum amplitudes of the strong transients are approximately 10 times larger than of the intermediate transients which are all less than one tick on the Volt axis in the figure. The signal leading and trailing the strong transients is a weak/intermediate signal. As can be observed upon comparing Figures 15(a) and 15(b) the approach is able to tackle the strong transients and identify them. It is interesting to notice that no transients are detected in the transient fluctuations during the decay of the large transient that starts at 11.6 ms. The transients in the decay manage to blend into each other so that they are not represented in the detection functions.

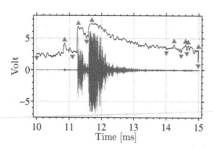

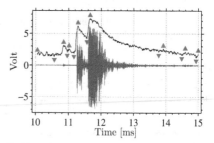

(a) The strong transients and the corresponding detection function in the time domain.

(b) The strong transients and the corresponding detection function in the time-frequency domain.

Figure 15. The figures show the strong transients, the detection functions in more detail. Also shown are the results from the peak-picking of the detection functions; i.e., the detected troughs and peaks.

6. Conclusion and future research

The approach presented in this chapter was designed to detect and determine AE hits in AE signals where conventional threshold-based hit detection is not suitable; i.e., using a fixed or a floating threshold. Fixed thresholds are set at the start of the monitoring; i.e., tuned to the noise level of the AE signal. As the material degrades and AE is generated by the cumulative damage, the AE signal level increases and the threshold cannot be used to detect individual hits. Furthermore, neither the fixed threshold nor the floating threshold can be used to distinguish between hits when a burst of strong, slightly overlapping AE is encountered. This type of burst is for example encountered during cyclic testing of assembled CFRP composites. In [13] it was generated by the rubbing of splinters. The overall strength of the AE increased during the test due to due to cumulated damage, but not noise. For this reason, a floating threshold was not suitable. Furthermore, because the strength of the AE emissions varied within each cycle, it was difficult to set the appropriate response time of the floating threshold. If the response was set too fast the threshold was affected by strong transients.

The transformation of the detection functions into the decibel scale is useful when the transducer cannot be placed at the location of damage and the AE signal suffers from high attenuation. Furthermore, the transformation produces a detection function that makes it possible to use one setting for automatic hit determination of both strong and weak hits.

The resolution of the approach can be fine tuned by adjusting the threshold, T_{tp}. This threshold is used to filter out small local troughs and peaks in the detection function. If a high resolution is required; i.e., to detect pulsations in the signal, then the time domain is the appropriate choice. This is both due to the computational cost and the inherent trade-off between the time and frequency resolution of the time-scale/time-frequency based approaches.

The presented approach has, intuitively, its own limitations. These include the tuning of the parameters used, the required computational load and associated time-lag. The hit determination in the time domain, using the envelope of the signal's energy, has a significantly lower computational load than the STFT-based determination in the time-frequency domain. Although it does not suffer from the time-frequency trade-off associated with the STFT, it will have a slight time-lag if the envelope is filtered; e.g., moving average filters. The main concern is the computational load but, not the time-lag. This is because the detection function and the peak-picking are only to detect the presence of transients. The final determination; i.e., deciding whether it is a hit or not, is performed using conventional threshold approaches. Hence, the exact timing of the peak-picking is not necessary.

Two detection functions were presented in this chapter and used. Numerous of other detection functions can of course be created. The detection functions can be created in the time domain as well as in the time-scale/time-frequency domains. In some instances transients are only separable in the time-scale/time-frequency domains, where wavelets and Cohen's class of time frequency representation (TFR) are used, respectively. Both approaches have been shown to provide a good representation of signals and for this reason, they have been receiving increasing attention in the recent years. The successful detection of transients, using either wavelets or Cohen's class of TFR depends strongly on the choice of the wavelet function and the distribution function, respectively.

Acknowledgements

The author wishes to acknowledge Össur hf. for both providing prosthetic feet for testing and access to their testing facilities. Furthermore the funding for the work presented was supported by grants from the University of Iceland Research Fund, the Icelandic Research Council Research Fund, the Icelandic Research Council Graduate Research Fund and Landsvirkjun's Energy Research Fund.

Author details

Rúnar Unnþórsson

University of Iceland, School of Engineering and Natural Sciences, Iceland

References

[1] Breckenridge, F. R. & Eitzen, D. G. [2005]. Acoustic Emission Transducers and Their Calibration, in P. O. Moore (ed.), *Acoustic Emission Testing*, 3rd edn, Vol. 6 of *Nondestructive testing handbook*, American Society for Nondestructive Testing, Inc., Columbus, pp. 51–60.

[2] Carlos, M. F. & Vallen, H. [2005]. Acoustic Emission Signal Processing, in P. O. Moore (ed.), *Acoustic Emission Testing*, 3rd edn, Vol. 6 of *Nondestructive testing handbook*, American Society for Nondestructive Testing, Inc., Columbus, pp. 153–154.

[3] Giordano, M., Calabro, A., Esposito, C., D'Amore, A. & Nicolais, L. [1998]. An acoustic-emission characterization of the failure modes in polymer-composite materials, *Composites Science and Technology* 58(12): 1923–1928.

[4] Green, E. R. [1998]. Acoustic emission in composite laminates, *Journal of Nondestructive Evaluation* 17(3): 117–127.

[5] Higo, Y. & Inaba, H. [1991]. General problems of AE sensors, *ASTM Special Technical Publication* (1077): 7–24.

[6] Holroyd, T. J. [2000]. *The Acoustic Emission & Ultrasonic Monitoring Handbook*, Machine & Systems Condition Monitoring Series, first edition edn, Coxmoor Publishing Company, Kingham, Oxford, UK.

[7] Kamala, G., Hashemi, J. & Barhorst, A. A. [2001]. Discrete-Wavelet Analysis of Acoustic Emissions During Fatigue Loading of Carbon Fiber Reinforced Composites, *Journal of Reinforced Plastics and Composites* 20(3): 222–238.

[8] Kim, H. C. & Park, H. K. [1984]. Laser interferometry system for measuring displacement amplitude of acoustic emission signals, *Journal of Physics D (Applied Physics)* 17(4): 673–5.

[9] Mouritz, A. P. [2003]. Non-destructive evalutation of damage accumulation, in B. Harris (ed.), *Fatigue in Composites*, Woodhead Publishing Ltd., Cambridge, pp. 242–266.

[10] Nayeb-Hashemi, H., Kasomino, P. & Saniei, N. [1999]. Nondestructive evaluation of fiberglass reinforced plastic subjected to combined localized heat damage and fatigue damage using acoustic emission, *Journal of Nondestructive Evaluation* 18(4): 127–137.

[11] Rizzo, P. & di Scalea, F. L. [2001]. Acoustic Emission Monitoring of Carbon-Fiber-Reinforced-Polymer Bridge Stay Cables in Large-Scale Testing, *Experimental Mechanics* 41(3): 282–290.

[12] Tsamtsakis, D., Wevers, M. & De Meester, P. [1998]. Acoustic Emission from CFRP Laminates During Fatigue Loading, *Journal of Reinforced Plastics and Composites* 17(13): 1185–1201.

[13] Unnthorsson, R. [2008]. *Acoustic Emission Monitoring of CFRP Laminated Composites Subjected to Multi-axial Cyclic Loading*, Phd., University of Iceland.

[14] Unnthorsson, R. [2012]. Identifying and Monitoring Evolving AE Sources, *in* W. Sikorski (ed.), *Acoustic Emission*, InTech. http://dx.doi.org/10.5772/31398.

[15] Unnthorsson, R., Runarsson, T. P. & Jonsson, M. T. [2007a]. Monitoring The Evolution of Individual AE Sources In Cyclically Loaded FRP Composites, *Journal of Acoustic Emission* 25(December-January): 253–259.

[16] Unnthorsson, R., Runarsson, T. P. & Jonsson, M. T. [2007b]. On Using AE Hit Patterns for Monitoring Cyclically Loaded CFRP, *Journal of Acoustic Emission* 25(December-January): 260–266.

[17] Unnthorsson, R., Runarsson, T. P. & Jonsson, M. T. [2008]. Acoustic Emission Based Fatigue Failure Criterion for CFRP, *International Journal of Fatigue* 30(1): 11–20. http://dx.doi.org/10.1016/j.ijfatigue.2007.02.024.

[18] Unnthorsson, R., Runarsson, T. P. & Jonsson, M. T. [2009a]. Acoustic Emission Feature for Early Failure Warning of CFRP Composites Subjected to Cyclic Fatigue, *Journal of Acoustic Emission* 26: 229–239. submitted.

[19] Unnthorsson, R., Runarsson, T. P. & Jonsson, M. T. [2009b]. AE Entropy for the Condition Monitoring of CFRP Subjected to Cyclic Fatigue, *Journal of Acoustic Emission* 26: 262–269.

[20] Vallen-Systeme GmbH [1998]. Product leaflet for integral Amplifier Transducers.

[21] Wevers, M. [1997]. Listening to the sound of materials: acoustic emission for the analysis of material behaviour, *NDT and E International* 30(2): 99–106.

[22] Ono, K. & Gallego, A. [2012]. Research and Applications of AE on Advanced Composites, Keynote paper, *The 30th European Conference on Acoustic Emission testing and 7th International Conference on Acoustic Emission*, pp. 4–47.

Chapter 2

Acoustic Emission Application for Monitoring Bearing Defects

Zahari Taha and Indro Pranoto

Additional information is available at the end of the chapter

1. Introduction

Several studies have been conducted to investigate AE application in bearing defects diagnosis and monitoring. The application of AE to measure the condition of slow speed antifriction bearings on off-shore gas production platform slewing cranes have been investigated by Rogers [1]. It was found that AE sensors can detect defects before they appeared in the vibration acceleration range and can also detect possible sources of AE generated during a fatigue life test of thrust loaded ball bearing [2, 3]. Morhain and David [4] showed the application of AE to monitor defects on the inner and outer races of split bearings.

Some researchers have studied AE based on the types of defects, locations, and various bearing operation condition. Smith and Fadden [5,6] identified the acoustic emission signals to detect defects in the form of a fine scratch on the inner race of axially loaded angular contact ball bearing at low speed only. The usefulness of some acoustic emission parameters, such as peak amplitude and count for detection of defects in radially loaded ball bearings at low and normal speed have been demonstrated [7].

Tan [8] suggested that, measurement of the area under the amplitude-time curve is a preferred method for detection of defects in rolling element bearings. Distribution of events by counts and peak amplitude has been used for detecting bearing defects [9]. Hawman and Galinaitis [10] noted that diagnosis of bearings defect is accomplished by high-frequency modulation of AE bursts at the outer race frequency.

The types of bearing used will affect the types of defects criteria to be simulated. Some researchers have used many types of bearings. Choudury and Tandon [11] have used the NJ series cylindrical roller bearing of normal clearance with five sizes of SKF bearing. NJ series bearings were chosen because the inner races of these bearings can be easily separated and thus the creation of simulated defects on the inner races and the rollers become easier. One simulated defect was introduced across the length of a roller bearing and the inner raceway by spark erosion technique. Cooper split-type roller bearing was selected with assembly and disassembly accomplished with minimum disruption to the test sequence. Two defect types used were surface discontinuity of the outer race and material protrusions that are clearly above the average surface roughness [12]. C.J Li and S.Y Li [13] used the ball bearing under four conditions: good bearing, a bearing with a groove on its outer race, bearing with a single roller defect, and a bearing with three outer race defects. The size of the artificial defects was 15.2 mm in diameter by 0.127 mm in depth and the width of the groove was 2 mm.

Choudury and Tandon [11] used the counts and statistical distribution of events by counts and peak amplitudes, and showed that as the defect size increases, more events are emitted with higher values of peak amplitudes and counts. It was also shown that the increase in counts is much greater than in other parameters, such us events and peak amplitudes. C.J Li and S.Y Li [13] showed that defects at different location of bearing (inner race, roller, and outer race) will have characteristic frequencies at which bursts are generated. The signal emitted by damaged bearing consists of periodic bursts of AE. The signal is considered to be amplitude modulated at the characteristic defect frequency.

Traditional techniques were used for detecting localized defects mainly based upon the processing of vibration and sound measured near the bearing with time domain techniques such as: peak level and r.m.s value [14], crest factor analysis [15], kurtosis analysis [16], and shock pulse counting [17]. Counts, events, and peak amplitude of the signal can be investigated and compared with each other to find more sensitive and accurate values.

In roller bearing application, the forces transmitted in the bearing give rise to stresses of varying magnitudes between the surfaces in both rolling and sliding motion. As a result of repeated loads concentrated contacts, changes occur in the contact surfaces and in the regions below the surfaces. These changes cause surface deterioration or wear [18]. The loss or displacement of material from the surface will cause wear. Material loss may be loose debris.

Mild mechanical wear
Adhesive wear
Smearing
Corrosive (tribochemical) wear
Plastic flow
Surface indentation
Abrasive wear
Surface distress
Pitting
Fatigue spalling

Table 1. Bearing Failure Classification Due to Wear [18]

Material displacement may occur by local plastic deformation or the transfer of material from one location to another location. When wear has reached the level that it threatens the essential function of the bearing, the bearing is considered to have failed. Bearing failures can be classified as in table 1.

In this research AE data is analyzed in the time domain. Peak amplitude, r.m.s., and AE counts were investigated and correlated with the type of defects, size of defect, speed, and applied load.

2. Experimental setup

A sketch of the rig on which the experiments were conducted is shown in figure 1. It consists of a shaft (2) supported on the base plate of a lathe machine and mounted on the chuck mounting. The bearing housing (5) supports the test bearing and is mounted on a base plate. The bearing housing is a plummer block housing type, SKF-SNL 516-513 series. Bolts, nuts, and washers are used to mount it on the base plate. Locating rings inside the housing restrict the movement of the shaft.

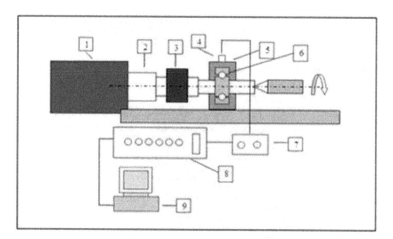

1. Motor driver, from spindle of Colchester lathe machine
2. Shaft
3. Load
4. AE sensor
5. Bearing housing
6. Test bearing
7. Piezotron AE Coupler
8. Signal Conditioning
9. PCI Data Acquisition (DAQ)

Figure 1. The experimental setup diagram

The shaft is extended beyond the right tailstock of the lathe machine such that the test bearing (6) may be easily mounted or dismounted from it. The extended portion of the shaft is stepped and of varying diameter to allow testing of different sizes of bearings and also to vary the load. The drive to test the rig is provided by the spindle of the lathe machine (1) and transmitted through a chuck mounted on the shaft. The speed of the rig can be adjusted easily by a variable control speed knob between the ranges 0 up to 3,250 rpm. To apply radial load on the test bearing a pulley load model is used (3). The pulley load is designed and calibrated to satisfy the load testing condition. The AE sensor (4) is mounted on the top of the test bearing housing by a magnetic clamp so that the measurement is performed in the nearest zone of the burst signal.

3. Test bearings and housing

The test bearings used in the study are self-aligning ball bearings from SKF series 1311 ETN9 with inside bore diameter 55 mm, outside diameter 120mm, and width 29 mm (figure 2). These bearings can self-align while operating inside the housing and also the inner race can be easily separated thus the creation of simulated defects on the inner races and rollers become easier.

The test bearing has a double row, consisting of 30 ball elements with 15 balls in each row. The bearing has dynamic and static load rating of 50.7 KN and 18 KN, respectively, a maximum speed rating of 7500 rpm, and weighs 1.6 kg. The appropriate bearing housing for the self-aligning ball bearing series 1311 ETN9 is the SNL 513-611 plummer block housing type from SKF. The housing encapsulates the test bearing and provide space for mounting the AE sensor. Figures 2 to 5 show the experimental set-up of the test bearings.

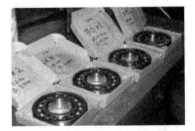

Figure 2. SKF Self aligning ball bearing used as test bearing

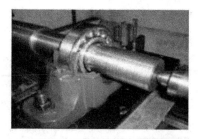

Figure 3. Test bearing arrangement on the housing, locating rings, and others equipments

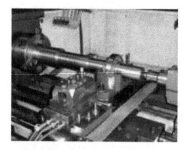

Figure 4. Shaft, test bearing, and the housing arrangement on the lathe machine

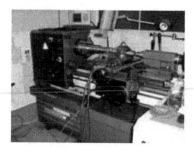

Figure 5. A view of the experimental set-up

4. Instrumentation

Measurements were carried out using an instrumentation system that consist of an AE sensor Kistler 8152 B121, an AE PZT coupler Kistler 5125B2, a DAQ card NI 6034 E, a BNC connector NI, signal conditioning SC 2345 NI, and Lab view software on a PCI system (Figures 6 to 8). The AE sensor has a frequency range of 50 – 400 kHz, 10 dB, sensitivity 57 dBref 1V/(m/s) and is mounted on the test bearing using a magnetic clamp from Kistler.

An AE PZT coupler with a gain process the high frequency output signals from the sensor and filter the signals. The gain can be set with a jumper. The frequency output of the coupler has an AE RMS output in a range of 10-1000 kHz and AE filtered output of 5-1700 kHz. The data acquisition NI 6034E series have 16 analog inputs at up to 200 kS/s, 16-bit resolution and Lab View 7.0 software is used for acquiring and processing the data. The AE PZT coupler is powered by a DC power supply with 0-2 A current range and 0-30 V voltage range.

5. AE sensor

In this research, the AE signal is obtained from an AE sensor. The sensor used is a Kistler AE sensor type 8152 B121. The sensor has an integral impedance converter for measuring AE above 50 kHz. With its small size it mounts easily near the source of emission to optimally capture the signal. The sensor has a very rugged welded housing (with degree of protection IP 65 PUR or IP 67 Viton).

The AE sensor consists of the sensor housing, the piezoelectric sensing element, and the built-in impedance converter. The sensing element is made of piezoelectric ceramic and mounted on a thin steel diaphragm. Its construction determines the sensitivity and frequency response of the sensor. The sensor have the capability of high sensitivity and wide frequency range, inherent high-pass-characteristic, insensitive to electric and magnetic noise field, and ground isolated to prevents ground loops. The sensor is mounted in the bearing housing with a magnetic clamp (figure 6)

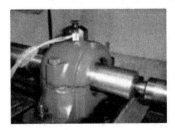

Figure 6. AE sensor mounting on the bearing housing with a magnetic clamp

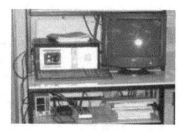

Figure 7. Instrumentation apparatus: PCI DAQ card, Connector block, and DC power supply

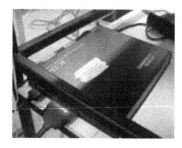

Figure 8. Data acquisition board signal conditioning SC-2345

6. AE–Piezotron coupler

The AE-Piezotron Coupler processes the high frequency output signal from AE sensor (Figure 9). Gain, filters, and integration time constant of the built-in-RMS converter are design as plug-in modules. This allows the best possible adaptation to the particular monitoring function. The gain can be set until 100 times. The amplifier has two series-connected second order filters, design as plug elements. The types of filter (high pass or low-pass) as well as the frequency limit are freely selectable.

A band pass filter is obtained by the series connection of one high-pass and one low-pass filter. The integration time constant of the RMS converter can also be freely selected. The limit switch is set with a potentiometer, and the switching threshold set point can be monitored at the limit output with an oscilloscope. The output of the limit switch is electrically isolated by an optocoupler. The output signals are available at the 8-pole round connector: two analog output signals AE output (Filter), AE-Out (RMS) and a Digital output signal (Limit Switch)

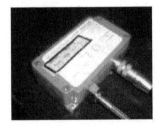

Figure 9. AE Piezotron Coupler Data Acquisition and Processing

6.1. PCI data acquisition board 6034E

Data acquisition system is implemented by a PCI 6034 E card. Data acquisition is performed using the Lab View 7.0 software and NI-DAQ Driver. The NI- DAQ has an extensive library of functions that can be called from an application programming environment. In this research, buffered data acquisition function is used as high speed A/D conversion process.

The NI-DAQ also has a high-level DAQ-I/O function for maximum capacity. The example of high-level function is streaming data to the hard disk or acquiring a certain number of data points. NI-DAQ maintains consistent software interface among its different version so that the platform can be changed with minimal modification to the software code.

In data acquisition application, there are many programs language that can be used. Zang illustrated the application of data acquisition developed using the NI-DAQ driver software and also show the relationship with other software and environment (Figure 10) [19].

6.2. Data acquisition and user interface

In this research, when monitoring the bearing defects, AE signal was captured using the Lab View Library. The data obtained was sampled using the windows XP interface to display the correlation graph and trend of AE signal. The Lab View 7 Software provides the Windows interface that makes the data processing more user friendly. Figure 11 describes the process of data acquisition and processing in this research.

7. AE counts and threshold level

The AE counts indicates the number of times the amplitude exceeds a preset voltage in a given times and gives a simple number characteristic of the signal. Many researchers have investigated the used of AE counts to detect defects on the bearing. Mba and Rao [9] stated that the successful use of AE counts for bearing diagnosis is dependent on the particular investigation, and the method of determining the trigger level is at the discretion of the investigator. They also stated that AE counts are also sensitive to the level and grade of lubricant within the bearing, adding the complexity of this measure.

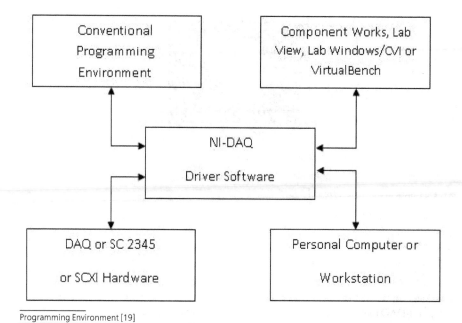

Programming Environment [19]

Figure 10. Relationship between the NI-DAQ Software and Hardware

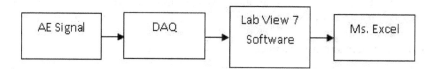

Figure 11. The schematic diagram of acquisition and processing the data

Morhain and Mba undertook an investigation to ascertain the most appropriate threshold level for AE counts diagnosis in rolling element bearings. The result shows that values of AE maximum amplitude did correlate with increasing speed but not with load and defect size. In addition, they stated that the relationship between bearing mechanical integrity and AE counts is independent of the chosen threshold level, although a threshold of at least 30% of the maximum amplitude for the lowest speed and load operating condition was suggested [4].

To calculate the AE counts from the defects, there are some parameters that have to be determined:

1. Maximum amplitude of background noise

2. The preset or threshold level as a reference to calculate the number of times the AE of defects exceed it.

The data processed from Lab View and Ms Excel gives the maximum amplitude of background noise and the defects. The characteristic of a maximum amplitude of AE is a burst signal, which is the maximum amplitude in the time domain graph that is not frequently distributed. Using the maximum amplitude as a reference of AE counts is not recommended.

Investigation of preset values in wide ranges of percentages of maximum amplitudes of background noise is useful to calculate the AE counts. The percentage levels of maximum amplitude are called threshold levels. The threshold levels ensure that the AE counts are calculated in wide ranges percentages of maximum amplitude of AE. Investigation of the AE counts in many threshold levels is useful to get the appropriate threshold levels range in real time monitoring.

In this study, the threshold levels were chosen as percentage of maximum amplitude of the corresponding background noise level. For example to calculate the AE counts for ball defect at 1500 rpm, the threshold level will be the percentage of the maximum amplitude of background noise at 1500 rpm (N15L0). In order to investigate the relationship between the threshold level and AE counts, five threshold values were calculated at varying percentages. The percentage values selected were 10%, 30%, 50%, 70%, and 90%. The wide ranges of values will be useful for determining the influence of threshold value on AE count result. The threshold levels for all rotational speed are show in table 2 below:

Threshold Value						
Noise Condition	Maximum Voltage (volt)	Amplitude Level (volt) for Each Percentage				
		10%	30%	50%	70%	90%
N3L0	0.6	0.06	0.18	0.30	0.42	0.54
N5L0	1.2	0.12	0.36	0.60	0.84	1.08
N7L0	1.8	0.18	0.54	0.90	1.26	1.62
N15L0	6.3	0.63	1.89	3.15	4.41	5.67
N30L0	18.15	1.82	5.45	9.08	12.71	16.34

Table 2. Threshold value for different noise condition

8. AE counts of ball defects

The number of AE counts for ball defect size 1 is shown in figures 12 to 16 below. Figures 17 to 21 show the number of AE counts for ball defect size 2.

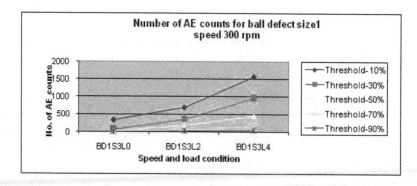

Figure 12. Number of AE counts for ball defect size 1 at speed 300 rpm

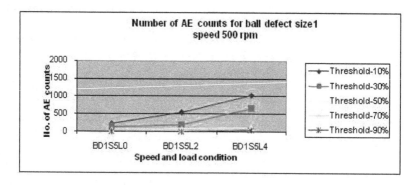

Figure 13. Number of AE counts for ball defect size 1 at speed 500 rpm

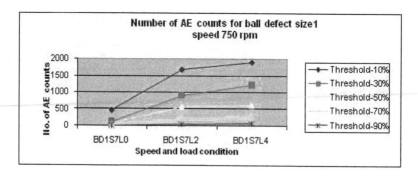

Figure 14. Number of AE counts for ball defect size 1 at speed 750 rpm

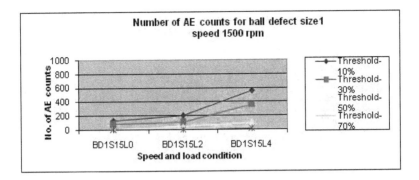

Figure 15. Number of AE counts for ball defect size 1 at speed 1500 rpm

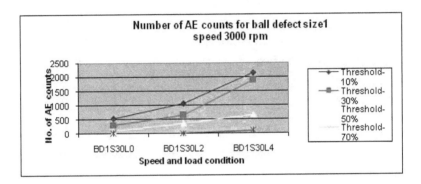

Figure 16. Number of AE counts for ball defect size 1 at speed 3000 rpm

From the result of AE counts in ball defect size 1, the value of AE counts increases with increasing load for all level of threshold. The increasing value is seen more clearly at percentages 50%, 30%, and 10%. This phenomenon is also observed from the result of AE counts in ball defect size 2, as shown in figures 17 to 21 below. The results also show that the number of AE counts of ball defect size 2 is greater than counts of size 1 for each respective rotational speed level and load. The graph for ball defect size 2 also indicates that, at percentages level of 50%, 30%, and 10% the AE counts clearly increases as the load increases.

In ball defect analysis, the result clearly showed that the AE counts increases with increasing load and size of defect at all rotational speed. The results are very clear at threshold level at or less than 50 % (50%, 30%, and 10%).

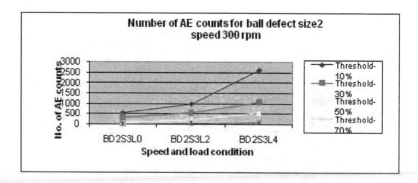

Figure 17. Number of AE counts for ball defect size 2 at speed 300 rpm

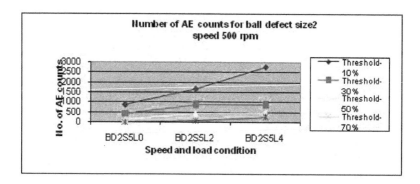

Figure 18. Number of AE counts for ball defect size 2 at speed 500 rpm

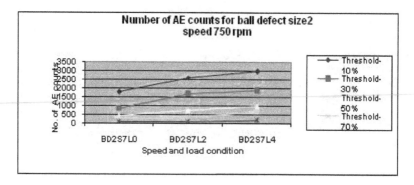

Figure 19. Number of AE counts for ball defect size 2 at speed 750 rpm

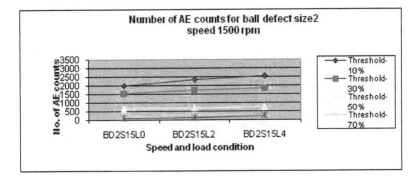

Figure 20. Number of AE counts for ball defect size 2 at speed 1500 rpm

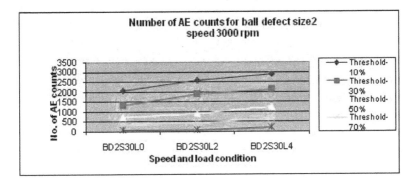

Figure 21. Number of AE counts for ball defect size 2 at speed 3000 rpm

9. AE counts of inner race defects

The number of AE counts for inner race defect size 1 are shown in figures 22 to 26 below and figures 27 to 31 show the number of AE counts for inner race defect size 2.

The result of AE counts in the inner race defect shows different phenomenon compared with the ball defect. For the inner race defect size 1, at 300 rpm and 500 rpm the AE counts increases as the load increases at threshold levels of 30% and 10%. Whilst at 750 rpm, 1500 rpm, and 3000 rpm the AE counts increases as load increases at 50%, 30%, and 10% threshold levels. In general the AE counts increases with increasing load.

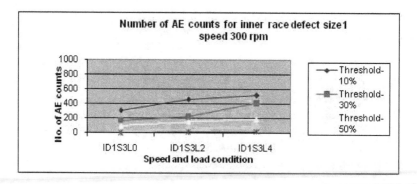

Figure 22. Number of AE counts for inner race defect size1 at speed 300 rpm

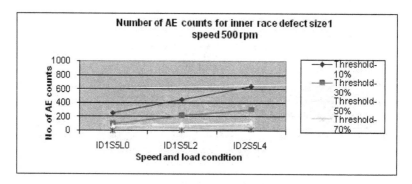

Figure 23. Number of AE counts for inner race defect size 1 at speed 500 rpm

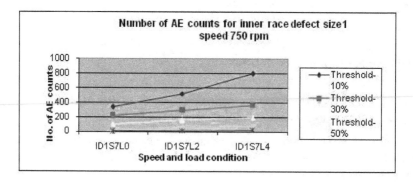

Figure 24. Number of AE counts for inner race defect size1 at speed 750 rpm

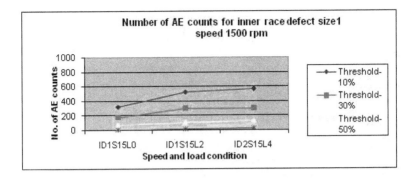

Figure 25. Number of AE counts for inner race defect size1 at speed 1500 rpm

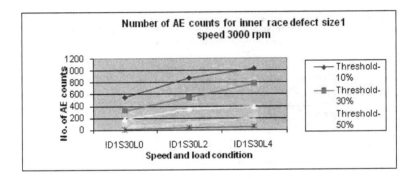

Figure 26. Number of AE counts for inner race defect size1 at speed 3000 rpm

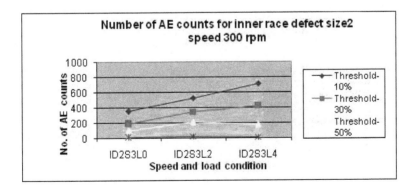

Figure 27. Number of AE counts for inner race defect size2 at speed 300 rpm

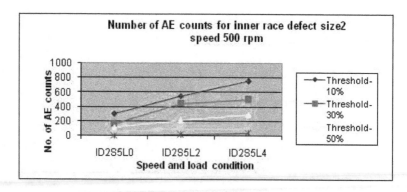

Figure 28. Number of AE counts for inner race defect size2 at speed 500 rpm

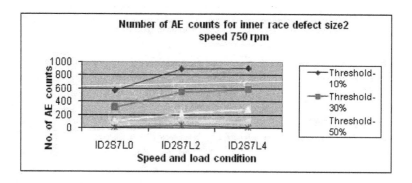

Figure 29. Number of AE counts for inner race defect size2 at speed 750 rpm

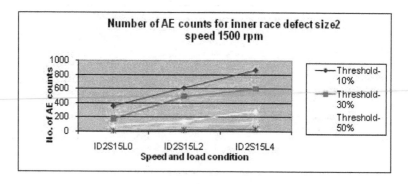

Figure 30. Number of AE counts for inner race defect size2 at speed 1500 rpm

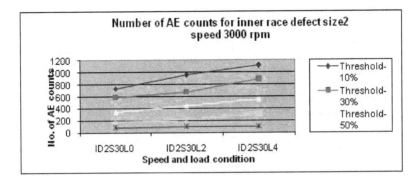

Figure 31. Number of AE counts for inner race defect size2 at speed 3000 rpm

For inner race defect size 2, at 300 rpm the AE counts increases as load increases at threshold levels of 30% and 10%. Whilst at 500 rpm and 750 rpm the AE counts increases as load increases at threshold levels of 50%, 30%, and 10%. And at 1500 rpm and 3000 rpm the AE counts increases as load increases at 70%, 50%, 30%, and 10% threshold levels. It is difficult to distinguish the AE counts of defect size 1 with defect size 2 for all respective speeds and threshold levels.

10. Conclusion

The results of the study shows AE counts can be used to detect defects in bearings. It also shows the correlation between the AE counts with speeds and loads. It is important to choose the appropriate range of threshold levels. A range of at least 30% (90%, 70%, 50%, 30%) of the maximum amplitude of the background noise was found to be effective..Morhain and Mba [4] stated that there isn't an ideal threshold level for all operating condition in bearing diagnosis, so investigation of background noise at all operational speed can be very useful. The use of AE r.m.s and counts is more successful for ball defects rather than inner race defects..

Author details

Zahari Taha[1] and Indro Pranoto[2]

1 Faculty of Mechanical Engineering, University Malaysia Pahang, Malaysia

2 Department of Mechanical and Industrial Engineering, Gadjah Mada University, Indonesia

References

[1] Roger LM, The application of vibration signature analysis and acoustic emission source location to on-line monitoring of antifriction bearing, Tribology International 12(2) (1979): 51-9

[2] Yoshioka T, Fujiwara T, New acoustic emission source locating system for the study of rolling contact fatigue, Wear 81(1) (1982):183-6

[3] Yoshioka T, Fujiwara T, Application of acoustic emission technique to detection of rolling bearing failure, American Society of Mechanical Engineers 14(1984): 55-76

[4] Morhain A, Mba D, Bearing defect diagnosis and acoustic emission, Journal of Engineering Tribology, Institution of Mechanical Engineering 217(4) (Part J) (2003) 257-272 (ISSN 1350-6501)

[5] Smith JD, Vibration monitoring of bearings at low speeds, Tribology International 1982; June: 139-44

[6] McFadden PD, Smith JD, Acoustic emission transducer for the vibration monitoring of bearings at low speeds, Proc. IMechE 198(C8) (1984):127-30

[7] Tandon N, Nakra BC, Defect detection in rolling element bearings by acoustic emission method, J Acoustic Emission 9(1) (1990): 25-8

[8] Tan CC, Application of acoustic emission to the detection of bearing failures, In: Proceeding, Tribology Conference, Brisbane, Australia: Institution of Engineers, 1990:110-4

[9] Bansal V, Gupta BC, Prakash A, Eshwar VA, Quality inspection of rolling element bearing using acoustic emission technique, J Acoustic Emission 9(2)(1990):142-6

[10] Hawman M.W., Galinaitis W.S., Acoustic emission monitoring of rolling element bearings, Proceedings of the IEEE, Ultrasonics Symposium (1988): 885-9

[11] Choudhury A, Tandon N, Application of acoustic emission technique for detection of defects in rolling element bearings, Tribology International 33 (2000): 39-45

[12] Abdullah M.A., David Mba, A comparative experimental study on the use of acoustic emission vibration analysis for bearing defect identification and estimation of defect size, Mech. System and Signal Processing J (2004): 1-35

[13] C. James Li, S.Y. Li, Acoustic emission analysis for bearing condition monitoring, Wear 185 (1995): 67- 74

[14] E. Downharm and R. Wood, The rationale of monitoring vibration on rotating machinery in continuously operating process plant, ASME Paper No.71- vibr-96

[15] B. Wiechbrodt and J. Bowden, Instrument for predicting bearing damage, GE company Rep., March, 1970, S-70-1021 AD 869633

[16] D. Dyer and R.M. Stewart, Detection of rolling element bearing damage by statistical vibration analysis, J. Mech (1978):229-235

[17] O.G. Gustafsson and T. Tallian, Detection of damage in assembled rolling bearings, Trans. Am. Soc. Lubric. Eng., 5 (1962):197-205

[18] Tedric A. Harris, Rolling Bearing Analysis, 4th Ed., John Wiley and Sons, Inc, USA, 2001

[19] Zhang Zhen, A Tool Condition Monitoring Approach Based on SVM, Master Thesis, National University of Singapore, 2002

Chapter 3

Acoustic Emission to Detect Damage in FRP Strength Under Freeze and Thaw Cycles

Hyun-Do Yun and Wonchang Choi

Additional information is available at the end of the chapter

1. Introduction

Strengthening with carbon fiber reinforced polymer (CFRP) sheets and plates, as opposed to the use of steel plates, has been employed recently in the rehabilitation and retrofitting of infrastructures due to better performance (than that of steel plates) in terms of resistance to corrosion and high stiffness-to-weight ratios. Because concrete structures are exposed periodically to snow and freezing temperatures during the winter season, a reduction in structural integrity, such as observed in the deterioration of the concrete and the degradation of the FRP bond system, is evident in field conditions. In terms of environmental exposure, periodic temperature changes such as freeze and thaw cycles can cause devastating damage to RC structures.

Since 1989, research by Kaiser [1] has been used to investigate the structural integrity of CFRP-strengthened RC beams exposed to freeze and thaw cycling. Results indicate that the strength of RC beams with CFRP sheets does not decrease with fewer than 100 cycles ranging from -25°C to 25°C. Similar test results are reported by Baumert and Bisby [2] who conducted tests on CFRP-strengthened RC beams exposed to temperatures ranging from -27°C to 21°C and from -18°C to 15°C with 50 freeze and thaw cycles for each temperature. Bisby and Green [3] examined the bonding performance of concrete members strengthened with CFRP and glass FRP under freeze and thaw cycling with temperatures ranging from -18°C to 15°C. Their results indicate insignificant effects on strengthening in flexure within 300 cycles of freeze and thawing. The American Concrete Institute (ACI) 440R-02 [4] recommends that the FRP system, which is exposed to high humidity, freeze-thaw cycles, salt water, or alkalinity, should be taken into account when determining the environmental degradation of an adhesively bonded system.

2. Problem statement

Because the condition of strengthened concrete is not visible from outside the CFRP sheets, it is difficult to quantify the deterioration and any defects that affect the structural integrity of the infrastructure. Evaluation techniques are needed to expand CFRP's application in repair and rehabilitation. With that need in mind, an acoustic emission technique is employed to determine the performance of CFRP-strengthened RC beams exposed to freeze and thaw cycling.

The author's previous study successfully shows the possible application of acoustic emission activities to determine the structural integrity corresponding to the representative damage levels of CFRP-strengthened RC beams that contain intentional defects in the bond system [5]. In this research, the acoustic emission signal characteristics of RC beams strengthened with CFRP sheets and exposed to several freeze and thaw cycles (0, 30, 60,120, and 400 cycles) ranging in temperature from -18 to 4°C are investigated.

For this study, six beams were fabricated in 100 x 100 x 400 mm sections with a specified design compressive strength of 33 MPa for all specimens. The specimens were designed in shear failure regardless of the shear reinforcement with CFRP. Specimen S1 indicates the control beam without any strengthening or freeze and thaw cycles. Specimens S2 indicate the shear-strengthened beams with CFRP sheets (0.12 mm thickness). Detailed reinforcement and specimen information is presented in Figure 1.

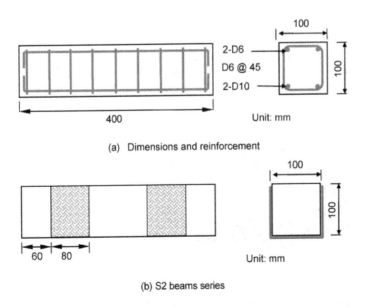

(a) Dimensions and reinforcement

(b) S2 beams series

Figure 1. Detailed information regarding the test specimens

The CFRP sheets used in this study have tensile strengths of 4,100 MPa, respectively. The adhesive (Sikadur-330) used for bonding the CFRP composites is epoxy resin, and its bonding strength, as supplied by the manufacturer, is 17.5 MPa. The material properties of the reinforcement in the specimens are listed in Table 1.

	Size of Rebar (diameter, area)	Yielding Strength (MPa)	Yielding Strain (μm)
Longitudinal Reinforcement	D13 (12.7mm, 1.267cm²)	255	2130
Transverse Reinforcement	D6 (6.35mm, 0.3167cm²)	290	1920
Compression Reinforcement	D6 (6.35mm, 0.3167cm²)	290	1920

Table 1. Material Properties of Reinforcement

The simply supported specimens were tested under four-point loading conditions by a 2000 kN Universal Testing Machine (UTM). The load was applied up to failure with displacement control of 0.1 mm/sec. Figure 2 shows the typical test set-up for the specimens used in this study. A linear variable differential transducer (LVDT) was installed to measure the displacement at the mid-span of the specimen. An electrical strain gauge also was installed to measure the strain in the tensile reinforcement and concrete. Four acoustic emission sensors (Model SE900-MWB with wide bandwidth) with a frequency range of 100~ 900 kHz were installed to measure the acoustic emission activities that correspond to the damage level of the specimens under flexure. These sensors were pre-amplified (at 20 dB) prior to recording in order to prevent noise signals due to friction, and a rubber sheet was placed between the beam and loading points. The threshold level was fixed to 35 dB to eliminate electric and mechanical noise. The acoustic emission signals were recorded up to the failure of the specimens.

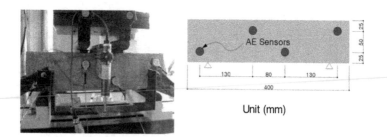

Figure 2. Typical test set-up and gauge installation

As the diagonal crack width expands, the specimen fails in shear mode, while multiple flexural cracks were generated for the S2 specimens with CFRP strengthening. For specimen

S1, the flexural crack initiates at the mid-span of the specimen around 12% (12 kN) of the ultimate strength, and then diagonal cracking is generated at around 30% (29kN) of the ultimate strength. As the diagonal crack width expands, the specimen fails in shear mode, while multiple flexural cracks were generated for the S2 specimens with CFRP strengthening.

As the load increases, the diagonal crack width increases, and then finally it fails in shear mode. Similar crack propagation was observed for all CFRP-strengthened specimens. As seen in Figure 3, the CFRP-strengthened specimens exposed freeze and thawing cycles partially de-bonded due to the deterioration of the interface between the concrete surface and adhesive.

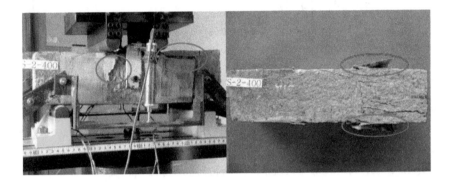

Figure 3. De-lamination of CFRP at failure

Figure 4 shows the load versus displacement relationship of the specimens. The CFRP-strengthened specimens prevent rapid strength reduction due to diagonal cracking once the ultimate strength is attained. The strength and ductility tend to decrease for the CFRP-strengthened specimens over 60 freeze and thawing cycles.

For the CFRP-strengthened specimen, the deformation in the diagonal direction rapidly increases. This occurrence results in the shear strengthening of the CFRP sheets. Moreover, the deformation in the diagonal direction increases as the number of freeze and thawing cycles increases. This occurrence results in the reduction of bond strength between the concrete surface and CFRP sheets.

2.1. Acoustic emission activities

2.1.1. Event counts and energy

Figure 5 shows the relationship between acoustic emission event counts and energy that corresponds to the normalized elapsed time (T/T_u). The normalized elapsed time is computed using the ratio of the loading time (T) to the moment of failure (T_u). The moment of failure is determined at the time of 80% ultimate strength after reaching the ultimate strength. Figure 5 show the rapid increase in the acoustic emission event counts at the initiation of flexural cracking. No external cracks or visible damage are evident prior to the initiation of the flexural cracks; however, a low level of events was recorded, which is possibly due to the voids and micro-cracks within the concrete.

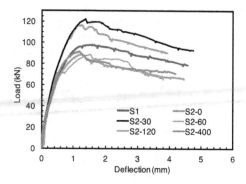

Figure 4. Load versus displacement

For specimen S1, the acoustic emission event counts moderately increase after the initiation of the flexural cracks.

For specimen S2, the acoustic emission event counts moderately increase after the initiation of the flexural cracks. Otherwise, the acoustic emission event counts for the CFRP-strengthened specimen, S2, increase and continue to increase along with the damage of adhesion in the interface between the concrete and CFRP plates.

The acoustic emission event counts for specimen S1 at the normalized elapsed time ratio of 41% drop within a short period due to the occurrence of diagonal cracks. Subsequently, the acoustic emission event counts increase up to the normalized elapsed time ratio of 64%, which is due to the incremental growth of the width of the existing diagonal crack, instead of the occurrence of a new crack. Compared with the occurrence of new cracks, increasing the width of existing cracks may result in a decrease in the occurrence of elastic waves [5].

Figure 5 show that the acoustic emission event counts for the specimens exposed to freeze and thaw cycles gradually increase from the beginning of the loading and continue to increase up to the ultimate loading. This occurrence may result in the weakness of the bond strength of the concrete within that causes deterioration of the structural integrity of the RC member. The acoustic emission energy tends to decrease gradually with an increase in the number of freeze and thaw cycles as shown in Figure 5.

The AE energy can be evaluated by the area of AE elastic waves. The AE energy level of the strengthened beam is higher energy level than that of the beam without strengthening. This was because the amplitude of AE signal due to the damage of epoxy is greater than that due to the crack in the concrete beam. The AE energy over 30 freeze and thawing cycles was rapidly increased. This was because the emitted AE elastic waves from the reduced bonding force between the CFRP sheets and epoxy were relatively lower than that from the rupture of epoxy which typically has a high level of amplitude characteristic.

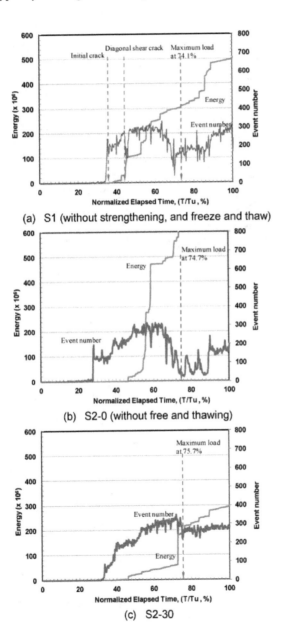

(a) S1 (without strengthening, and freeze and thaw)

(b) S2-0 (without free and thawing)

(c) S2-30

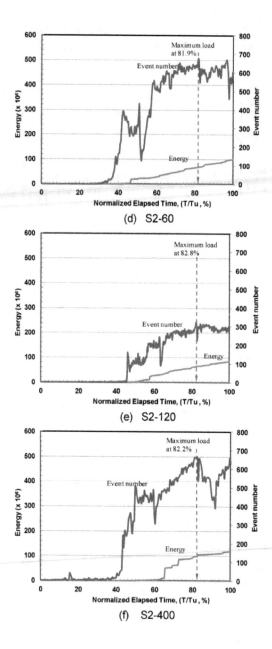

Figure 5. Acoustic emission event counts and energy characteristics of RC beams with CFRP composites (up to 0.80P$_{max}$ after maximum loading)

2.2. Amplitude and frequency

Figure 6 shows the progress of amplitude and frequency that corresponds to the normalized loading ratio for selected specimens. The amplitude and frequency of specimen S1 increase considerably from the beginning of the load to the initial flexural crack, as shown in Figure 6 (a). This result is caused by the development of macro-cracks that represent the connection of the voids and entrapped air within the concrete. The incremental development of the macro-cracks continues until diagonal cracks begin to appear. The frequency decreases radically once these diagonal cracks appear. However, the amplitude does not change significantly. The frequency decreases continuously until the ultimate load is reached. Afterward, it is in the range of 100 – 200 kHz until failure.

For specimen S2, the acoustic emission signal is detected at the beginning of loading. Specimen S2 generates a higher amplitude and frequency than specimen S1. These higher acoustic emission signals might be caused by the damage of epoxy on the concrete surface and CFRP plate. No considerable change is evident from the beginning of the de-bonding of the CFRP to the ultimate loading and failure. The frequency until failure is in the range of 150 – 250 kHz, which is a higher frequency than for specimen S1. This finding is due to the acoustic emission signal characteristics of the epoxy in the interface between the concrete and CFRP sheets.

On the other hand, specimens S2-120 and S2-400 generate low amplitude and frequency at the initial flexural cracks and diagonal cracks. This occurrence results in the deterioration of the epoxy and/or the concrete surface due to the considerable number of freeze and thawing cycles.

As shown in Figure 8 (f), the more freeze and thawing cycles, the more deterioration of the concrete surface and CFRP sheets. This deterioration results in the significant increase in amplitude and frequency during the beginning of loading up to the de-bonding of the CFRP. Afterward, the acoustic emission signal decreases. The frequency until failure is in the range of 200 – 350 kHz, which is a relatively high frequency range. In general, there is a tendency for the amplitude and frequency to increase as the micro-cracks and initial flexural cracks develop. The frequency tends to decrease as the diagonal cracks propagate and the crack widths expand, although the maximum amplitude does not change.

2.3. Damage evaluation

In order to apply acoustic emission techniques to the evaluation of damage and integrity of CFRP-strengthened RC beams, it is essential to study the characteristics of the acoustic emission parameters according to damage levels. The evolution of acoustic activity caused by micro-fracture within the concrete is often quantified using the concise framework originated by Gutenberg and Richter in their analysis of earthquake magnitudes, which is a reflection of the view that large-scale (i.e., geological) and small-scale (i.e., micro-fracture) acoustic events share a common origin in cascades of strain energy release events. In earthquake seismology, events of larger magnitude occur less frequently than events of smaller magnitude. This fact can be quantified in terms of a magnitude-frequency relationship, for which Gutenberg and Richter propose the empirical formula (1),

$$\log N(W) = a - bW,$$

(1)

where $N(W)$ is the Richter magnitude of the events, which is the cumulative number of events having a magnitude greater than or equal to W, and a and b are the empirical constants.

In acoustic emission data analysis, the coefficient b is known as the AE-b value [6]. The AE-b value is given as the gradient of the linear descending branch of the cumulative frequency distribution. The coefficient 20 was multiplied to get the AE-b values to the slope [7]. In the process where micro-fractures are more prevalent than macro-fractures, the b-value tends to increase, whereas in the process whereby macro-fractures occur more frequently than micro-fractures, the b-value tends to decrease.

Figure 7 presents the relationship of maximum amplitude versus frequency during the specific normalized elapsed time, which indicates the representative damage level. For specimen S2-120, the AE-b value is 1.389 when the micro-cracks initiate on the surface and can be detected visually. As the cracks propagate and expand, the values are 1.222 and 1.051, respectively. Those values tend to decrease as damage progresses. In short, the AE-b values tend to increase when the micro-cracks dominate the overall behavior, whereas the AE-b values seem to decrease when the behavior is controlled primarily by the propagating and expanding cracks [6, 8].

Figure 8 presents the comparison between the AE-b values versus the normalized elapsed time to failure. For specimen S-1, the AE-b value decreases significantly at the initiation of the diagonal cracks and flexural compression failure, at which time considerable damage is generated. This occurrence results in a high acoustic emission signal.

For specimen S-2, the lowest AE-b value is obtained at the de-bonding of the CFRP. Afterward, the rapid decrease in the AE-b value can be observed around the point of failure.

Specimens with fewer than 120 freeze and thawing cycles have relatively higher AE-b values (higher than 1.2) at the initiation of the micro-cracks and diagonal cracks and de-bonding of the CFRP. In general, the AE-b values range from 1.20 to 1.45, which is a relatively narrow fluctuation range compared to that for the specimens that are not exposed to freeze and thawing cycles.

For specimens exposed over 400 freeze and thawing cycles (S2-400), the low AE-b values are obtained at the beginning of the elapsed time, which may result in the deterioration of the concrete surface and bonding surface with the CFRP. The damage level caused by the freeze and thawing cycles is comparable to that of the macro-cracks. This occurrence is caused by the low acoustic emission values at the beginning of the test.

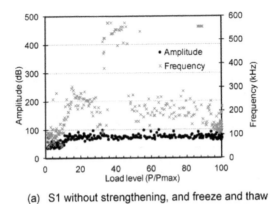

(a) S1 without strengthening, and freeze and thaw

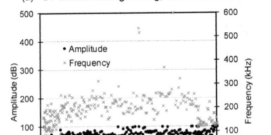

(b) S2 without free and thawing

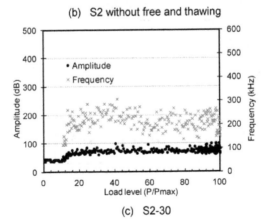

(c) S2-30

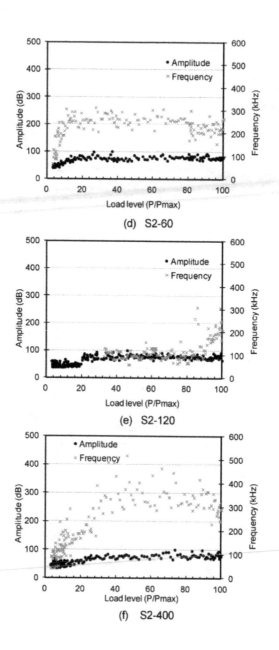

Figure 6. Frequency and amplitude

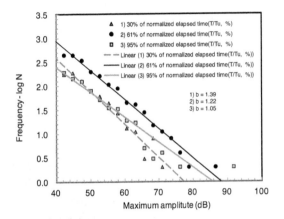

Figure 7. Typical variations of amplitude and load for S2-120

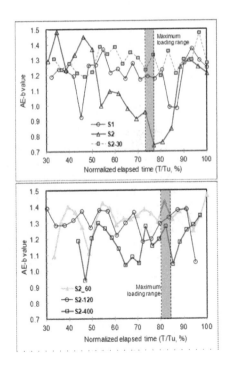

Figure 8. The AE-b values versus the normalized elapsed time to failure

In order to quantify the evolution of the damage process during the loading of the CFRP-strengthened RC beams, the AE-b values are separated into three subpopulations representing each damage level (i. micro cracks; ii. crack propagation and/or crack growth; iii. macro cracks; de-bonding, and/or CFRP failure). The relationship between the physical damage level and the AE-b value is presented in Table 2.

Range of AE-b values	Damage description
AE-b values "/> 1.25	Development of micro-crack
1.25 "/> AE-b values "/> 1.15	Propagation of micro-crack and crack width
1.15 "/> AE-b values "/> 0.80	Formation of macro-crack, de-bonding of CRFP, rupture

Table 2. AE-b Values for Each Damage Level

3. Conclusions

The strengthening performance and evaluation of the damage caused by acoustic emission activities for RC beams strengthened in shear with CFRP are examined under various freezing and thawing cycles with and without shear strengthening. The following results are found based on the limited experimental tests.

The significant increase in acoustic emission activities (event, energy, amplitude, and frequency) is observed at each damage level that corresponds to the initiation of the crack, propagation of diagonal cracking, de-bonding of CFRP, and failure. These acoustic emission activities are good indicators for determining the structural integrity and micro-damage of CFRP-strengthened RC beams.

The AE-b value provides a possible application to quantify the local damage of CFRP-strengthened RC beams exposed to freeze and thaw cycling corresponding to various damage levels.

Author details

Hyun-Do Yun[1] and Wonchang Choi[2]

1 Chung-Nam National University, Korea

2 NC A&T State University, USA

References

[1] Kaiser, H. P. Strengthening of Reinforced Concrete with Epoxy-Bonded Carbon Fibre Plastics. Doctoral thesis. Eidgenossische Technische Hochschule (ETH), Zurich: Switzerland; 1989.

[2] Baumert, M. E., M. F. Green, and M. A. Erki. Proceedings of the Second ACMBS International Conference, August11-14, 1996, Montreal, Canada.

[3] Bisby, L. A. and M. F. Green. Resistance to Freezing and Thawing of Fiber-Reinforced Polymer Concrete Bond. ACI Structural Journal 2002; 99(2) 215-223.

[4] ACI 440. Guide for the Design and Construction of Externally Bonded FRP systems for Strengthening Concrete Structures. 2002.

[5] Yun, H., W. Choi, and S. Seo. Acoustic Emission Activities and Damage Evaluation of Reinforced Concrete Beams Strengthened with CFRP Sheets. NDT & E International, Elsevier, 2010; 43(7) 615-628.

[6] Shitotani, T., Y. Nakanishi, X. Luo, and H. Haya. Damage Assessment in Railway Sub-structures Deteriorated Using Acoustic Emission Technique, DGZFP-Proceedings BB 90-CD, 2004.

[7] K. Mogi, Study shocks caused by the fracture of heterogeneous materials and its relations to earthquake phenomena, Bulletin of Earthquake Research Institute, University of Tokyo,1962; 40 123-173.

[8] Colombo, I. S., I. G. Main, and M. C. Forde. Assessing Damage of Reinforced Concrete Beam Using b-value Analysis of Acoustic Emission Signals. Journal of Materials in Civil Engineering, ASCE, 2003; 15(3) 280-286.

Chapter 4

Acoustic Emission in Drying Materials

Stefan Jan Kowalski, Jacek Banaszak and
Kinga Rajewska

Additional information is available at the end of the chapter

1. Introduction

Drying of wet materials is one of the oldest and most common unit operation found in diverse processes such as those used in the agricultural, ceramic, chemical, food, pharmaceutical, pulp and paper, mineral, polymer, and textile industries. It is also one of the most complex and least understood operations because of the difficulties and deficiencies in mathematical descriptions of the phenomena of simultaneous – and often coupled and multiphase – transport of heat, mass, and momentum in saturated porous materials. Drying is therefore an amalgam of science, technology, and art, or know-how based on extensive experimental observations and operating experience [Strumiłło, 1983; Mujumdar (Ed.), 2007].

Drying processes ought to be appropriately arranged and operated to obtain a high quality dried products, that is, products without excessive deformations, surface cracks, and above all crosswise fractures. A non-uniform moisture distribution in products arising during drying causes a non-uniform material shrinkage and generates stresses, which are responsible for permanent deformations and material fracture. A risk of fracture in drying samples is possible to analyze both theoretically and experimentally. Mechanistic drying models make the basis for numerical simulations of drying kinetics and analysis of the drying induced stresses [Kowalski, 2003]. In this way it is possible to determine the spots, where the drying induced stresses reach maximum and the possibly crack may occur [Kowalski and Rybicki, 2007]. The theoretical predictions are confronted with the experimental data obtained due to application of the acoustic emission method (AE), which enables monitoring *on line* the development of the drying induced fractures caused by stresses [Kowalski et al., 2000].

The acoustic emission method (AE) is a non-destructive method allowing indirect control of micro- and macro-fracture development during drying and above all the identification of the period and also the place where the fractures start to develop. In this sense the AE is a method that enables control of drying process and help to protect the material against destruction [Kowalski, 2010]. Thus, the EA provides a unique advantage of early detection of subcritical crack growth and recognize when and where the crack is growing. The cracks and deformations arising inside dried materials constitute the AE source. The intensity of AE signals, their number and energy inform about the state and magnitude of stresses [Kowalski, (2002), Kowalski et al., (2004)].

The aim of this chapter is to show the possibly using the AE method to diagnostic purposes of destruction due to monitoring materials subjected to drying. The results of the tests obtained from convective and microwave drying of ceramic and wood materials carried out in the laboratory drier equipped with the acoustic emission set-up constitute the illustrative material of this chapter.

The example under analysis concern cylindrical samples made of kaolin and wood. Based on the mechanistic drying model, the stress distribution in the samples and its evolution in time were determined. In this way the moment at which the stresses reach the critical value causing material damage was appointed [Kowalski et al. 2012]. The system of double coupled differential equations of this model, adopted to the cylindrical geometry, was solved numerically with the help of the finite element (FEM) and the finite difference (FDM) methods. Due to AE method, the number and the energy of AE hits were measured, and the crest value of acoustic waves was appointed, and these data enabled validation of the theoretical predictions. A good adherence of the theoretical and experimental results serves for identification of fractures occurring in materials during drying.

2. The essence of acoustic emission (AE) in drying

2.1. AE descriptors

- Different regimes of compresional acoustic waves propagating through the material from the crack places to the AE detectors attached to the samples, can be identified through the proper choice of the AE descriptors. The descriptors suitable to assessment of mechanical phenomena occuring in drying materials are selected mostly to be: *the number of acoustic emission hits*, *hit rate* (showing the dynamic of the process), *the maximum energy of hits*, and *the crest value* (showing the power of AE signals).

- When applying the AE method to drying processes, a suitable selection of AE descriptors that let to obtain the most useful information about the phenomena occurring in dried materials is an important issue. The parameters characterizing the AE signals that are recorded by the detector inform about intensity and possible size of destruction, and therefore are significant for the precise assessment of the AE occurrence. So, the appointing of the descriptors which qualitatively fit best for description of the AE occurrence is a responsible and difficult task.

- Based on the authors' experience and the performed up to now experiments, it was stated that AE descriptors best reflecting the character of mechanical phenomena occurring in drying materials, are:

- *Hits rate.* This descriptor shows the dynamics of the destruction development (e.g. a rise of temperature drying involves rapid growth of the AE hits rate). Moreover, this descriptor indicates the stages of drying, in which the reduction or increase of the AE activity takes place.

- *The hit of maximum energy.* This descriptor is more useful than that "energy of hits" as it shows the single hit with maximum energy in a given time interval. The descriptor "energy of hits" presents the energy of all hits in a given time interval.

- *Crest value.* This descriptor presents the intensity of hits in time. It is a very significant parameter illustrating the "power" of existing hits.

- *The total number of hits and the total energy of hits.* These parameters show some individual phenomena occurring during drying. Thanks to these descriptors it is possible to distinguish stages of drying in which some irregular changes of the AE energy or the AE hits rate appear. These descriptors point out the critical moments of drying, in which the fracture of drying material may occur.

2.2. Calibration of AE energy

The registered by the equipment AE signals are characterized by two fundamental parameters: the amplitude and the time of signal duration. The relative energy of each signal, called also the acoustic energy of AE signal, is possible to determine integrating the surface under the envelope curve of this signal. It is a relevant characteristics of the magnitude and power of the AE signal source. By application of the AE method to monitoring of drying processes, which are characterized with constant reduction of moisture content (MC) in dried materials, it should be taken into account that the AE energy depends on the material MC. If assume that the sources of AE signals cause cracks of a similar size, however, occurred first in wet material and next in dry one, then, the registered by the equipment AE signals will be different for these two events. This follows from damping of the acoustic waves propagating though a not perfectly elastic material. It is obvious that a more saturated material characterizes with stronger damping properties than an unsaturated one. Therefore, it is essential to take into account the damping effects by analysis of the AE energy descriptors.

It is necessary then to carry out the calibration of the AE energy for each examined material in dependence on its MC. There is a number of calibration methods (Malecki and Ranachowski 1994, Banaszak and Kowalski 2010). Here, the mechanical method is presented, that is, the method of falling ball (Berlinsky at al. 1990, Luong Phong 1994). The calibration was carried out with the use of the equipment presented in figure 1.

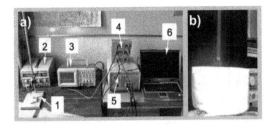

Figure 1. AE energy calibration set-up: a)1 – the ball's releasing mechanism and AE sensor, 2 – AC power supplier, 3 – oscilloscope, 4 –preamplifier, 5 – AE acquisition system AMSY5, 6 – computer, b) impact of dropping ball at the upper kaolin sample surface

A still ball of mass m = 5.60 g and diameter d = 11 mm was used as a source of acoustic signals having known and constant energy. The ball was planted in the grip with release mechanism, being the electromagnet connected to the power supply adaptor of direct current (2). The ball was situated at height of 10 cm above the upper surface of the sample. The AE sensor (1) was attached to the bottom surface of the sample. The registered AE signals were conveyed through the preamplifier (4) to the module unit AMS-5, where they were processed by means of control unit (6). The digital oscilloscope (3) was connected to the system to analyze the course of signal appearance and to assign the level of noise.

The release from the grip ball hit the upper surface of the sample (Fig. 1b) and generated elastic wave, which experienced damping when propagating through the not perfectly elastic sample. After its arriving to the AE sensor, it became converted into the electric signal and next undergone a suitable energetic analysis. Each test was repeated five times for each sample of given MC, and the average value was taken for further considerations. On the basis of those tests the curve of attenuation of the AE energy was determined as a function of the material MC. Figure 2 presents the results of the research carried out for the kaolin and the walnut wood.

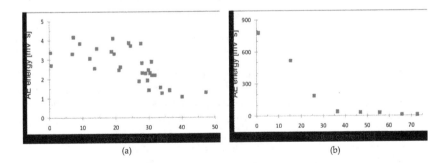

Figure 2. Damping of EA energy in dependence of material MC determined in the test of falling ball: a) kaolin, b) walnut wood

Damping of the AE signal energy depends strictly on the material moisture content. Kaolin material becomes plastic for the moisture content over 27-29% and thus it stronger attenuate the AE signals than that unsaturated one. For the walnut wood the attenuation of acoustic waves becomes very strong for the moisture contents above the fiber saturation point (FSP) (ca. 30%), and there remain on a constant level. Dry wood is a very acoustic material and the energy of AE signal in such a material is weakly attenuated. Alongside with the increase of the MC up to the fiber saturation point the damping of EA waves increases radically. Over this critical MC wood stops to be acoustic material and utters characteristic hollow sounds. It should be noted a very intensive linear drop of energy in the range below the fiber saturation point, what means that wood is a material very sensitive to changeability of the moisture content, for example, music instruments made of wood should be always adjusted to the actual air humidity.

There is a necessity of suitable correction of the energetic values of AE signals received from the measurement set-up, dependent on the actual MC of the material. For this purpose it is necessary to construct the calibration curve of AE energy for the tested material. It can be constructed by the best adjustment of the theoretical curve expressed by the fourth order polynomial to the experimental data. (Fig. 2).

Figure 3 presents the results of measurements of the mean energy of AE events for kaolin and walnut wood during drying with and without taking into account the calibration curve.

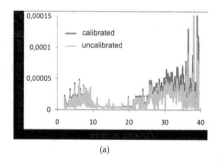
(a)

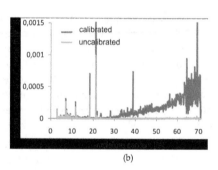
(b)

Figure 3. Comparison of mean energy of a AE hits as the function of material MC with and without taking into account of the damping effects during drying: a) kaolin, b) walnut wood

The curve of calibrated AE energy for kaolin has not a significant impact on the final results by the analysis of the AE events. The character of plots with and without taking into account the calibration curve is similar. It follows from insignificant difference in AE signal attenuation for saturated and unsaturated materials. For walnut wood, however, at the beginning of drying (ca. 70% MC) there were registered low energetic AE signals only. High energetic signals appear else by about 20% MC. Taking into consideration the fact that wood strongly attenuates the AE signal with increase MC, then, it can be noticed (Fig. 3b) that the real annotated AE energy, measured with using calibration curve, is significantly higher. It influences then the analysis of AE signals for MC above the fiber saturation point (30%). Some signals arriving to the AE sensor are high energetic ones even for MC 70% to 60%. The initial high energetic signals for such a high MC originate from sample heating. For example, the AE signal registered for 39% MC originates from a crack in the sample. This AE event could be identified else after taking into account in the analysis the calibration curve presenting the effects of AE energy damping. The other high energetic signals, connected with the successive cracks in the sample, were registered for the sample with MC below the fiber saturation point. They are clearly visible both for the calibrated and not calibrated energy with respect to the material MC.

The presented above results show how important is taking into account the damping of AE signals in studies of drying processes in which the AE method is used for monitoring of the mechanical effects, particularly in wood. Without such an approach a part of the AE signals can be wrongly interpreted, for example, some crack occurrence could not be noticed.

3. Experimental setup equipped with AE measurement instruments

3.1. Scheme of the equipment

The drying tests were realized in the laboratory hybrid drier in the Department of Process Engineering, Institute of Technology and Chemical Engineering, Poznań University of Technology. Presented in this chapter experimental results has been taken for over a decade and according to technical progress our measurement instruments obviously has changed few times during those years. Figure 4 presents the photograph of the latest dryer version equipped with the acoustic emission (AE) system.

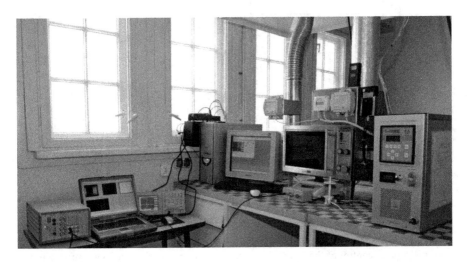

Figure 4. Photo of the laboratory hybrid dryer

Figure 5 presents the scheme of the dryer. The cylindrical kaolin or wood samples were placed in the drier chamber on a special ceramic thimble with mandrel embedded on the balance located beyond the chamber. In this way the measurement of the sample weight was possible continuously during all kinds of drying, also during microwave drying. The AE detector was attached either directly to the sample foundation by convective drying or indirectly to the ceramic thimble with mandrel by microwave drying.

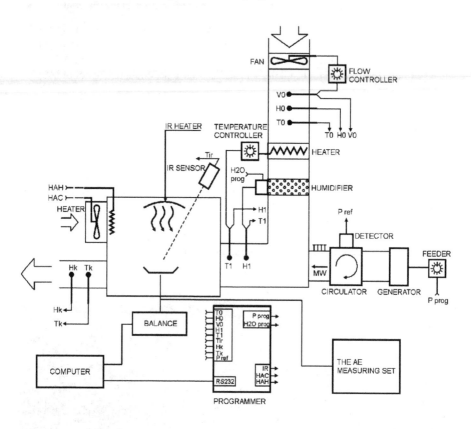

Figure 5. Scheme of the hybrid dryer

The hybrid drier enabled different combination of the three methods of drying: the convective, microwave, and infrared. The drier instrumentation enable programming and control of the velocity and temperature of the air supplied to the drier chamber, control of the microwave power, two-step control of the infrared heater, and the measurement of the sample surface temperature with the help of the optical pyrometer

3.2. Methodology of AE measurement

The AMSY-5 AE system manufactured by Vallen Systeme, Gmbh is shown in figure 4. The sample subjected to convective drying was placed on the aluminum plate with fixed piezo-electric sensor. Acoustic signals generated in the drying sample are registered by broad-band transducer. Next the signals were send via insulated cable to AEP3 preamplifier unit. Pream-plifiers was located close to AE sensors. The main task of preamplifier was amplifying and strength the signals enough that they could be sent to the distant main measurement unit. The AEP3 unit was equipped with 5 kHz to 1000 kHz filters. The main unit used in the tests had an M6 master unit for up to six AE channels from which three were fully equipped with ASSIP card. This high speed system could store up to 30 000 AE signals per second. The frequency filter inside the unit was used to eliminate noise sources. It can be set up for each channel separately. In our tests the low and high filters in the range from 12 to 850 kHz were applied to collect AE signals from kaolin and wood samples subjected to drying. The filtered AE signals were digitalized in A/D converter and stored in computer memory. The companion notebook PC had a software to control the whole measure system. During the tests the measured data were analyzed online and displayed on computer monitor so that it was possible to recognize the development of defects within the tested object.

4. Materials and conditions for AE appearance

KOC kaolin-clay from the Surmin-Kaolin SA Company, Nowogrodziec, Poland was the material investigated experimentally and theoretically in the drying tests. For this material some charakteristic data necessary for numerical calculation of drying kinetics and drying induced stresses were already given by the Surmin-Kaolin SA Company (see Table 1 in Kowalski et al. 2000). The KOC kaolin-clay is widely applied in ceramic industry for manu-facturing sanitaryware and tableware. It provides a good strength and plasticity during shaping of the mentioned products and reveals a reduced amount of pyroplastic deformation in the process of their firing.

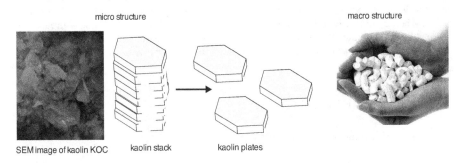

micro structure   macro structure

SEM image of kaolin KOC   kaolin stack   kaolin plates

Figure 6. Image of kaolin KOC

The kaolin-clay was delivered in a dry state, and before experiments it was grinded and wetted with a predetermined amount of water and mixed to achieve a greasy paste of initial moisture content (MC) approximately equal to 0.45 [kg water/kg dry kaolin]. The greasy paste was stored and homogenized in a closed box for 48 hours to unify moisture distribution in the whole material. The obtained in such a way soft kaolin-clay mass was used to mold cylindrical samples of 6 cm in diameter and 6 cm height. The cylindrical samples were extruded from a special instrument to preserve their regular shape (Fig. 7a), and samples of such a form were used for drying tests.

Figure 7 shows the shape of kaolin and pine wood samples applied in the studies.

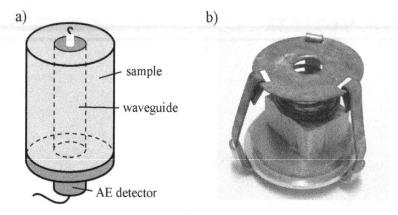

Figure 7. Image of the samples used in drying tests: a) kaolin cylindrical sample with attached AE detector, b) pine wood sample with spring pressed the sample to the AE detector

Samples of the pine wood in the form of cuboid of dimensions about 4×4×2 cm were cut from the blade of the trunk of diameter about 30 cm and keep the symmetry with regard to the axis of the core. The walnut samples were of cylindrical form with height about 26 ÷ 27 mm and the diameter about 44 ± 2 mm. These samples were cut out from walnut branches deprived of defects in the structure. They contained 5 annual growth rings on average. The samples were placed on the aluminum support to which they were pressed with the springs to get a better contact with the AE sensor. The initial humidity of pine wood samples was about 117% and walnut samples about 85%. The samples prepared in this way were used to convective and microwave drying tests in the laboratory dryer presented above.

5. Examples of AE in drying materials

5.1. Convective drying of ceramic-like materials

One of the goals of the realized tests was to interpret the AE signals that may occur during drying of kaolin-clay (Fig. 8). The first (I) characteristic group of AE signals appears at the beginning of drying process, the second (II) one in the period when the surface layer intensively shrinks, and third (III) one is noticeable sometimes in the final stage of drying and identified as being generated by the reversed stresses.

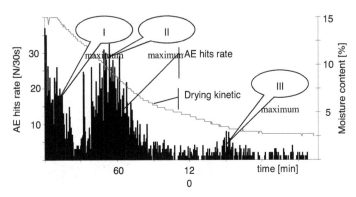

Figure 8. AE signals and the curve of drying

As the drying body is almost fully saturated at the initial stage of drying, the number and the maximum value of AE signals in the heating period (I) is proportional to temperature of the drying process. At this stage of drying, the thermal stresses dominate in the clay sample which are rather not so much meaningful. Unfortunately, at the initial stage of drying some of AE signals come from heating aluminium probe and the AE sensor. It is hard to decide which AE signals in this stage of drying are from the investigated kaolin-clay sample and which from other sources. In tests with lower process temperatures the first maximum was also lower.

The second group of AE signals is evidenced at the end of the constant drying period (II). Their number is the highest of the whole drying process. The reason for appearance of these signals can be explained by the tensional stresses that arise at the external layers of the cylinder as a result of shrinkage. The surface of the body becomes more and more dry while its core is kept still wet. The first cracks on the external surface of the cylinder are observed when the local stress reaches the yield strength or the strain exceeds the allowable ultimate limit.

The third (III) maximum of AE signals is rather of small or moderate magnitude and depends on drying conditions. It was stated that this maximum exists usually for high temperature or low humidity of the drying medium. It holds for porous materials revealing inelastic properties (e.g. wet wood, clay, kaolin), and can be explained as follows: at the beginning of drying, the external layers are stressed in tension and the core in compression. Inelastic strains occur both in the surface layer and in the wet core. Later, under a surface layer with reduced shrinkage, the core dries and attempts to shrink causing the stress state to reverse. These new induced tensional stresses in the core cause fracture of a brittle (almost dry) structure, in what follows generate the acoustic signals.

Fig. 9 presents the rate of AE hits for the five different temperatures of drying. It is seen that for the conditions of high drying rates created by high temperatures, the rate of AE hits achieve higher values than for lower temperatures. That high active emission of AE signals has a reflection in the drying induced stresses.

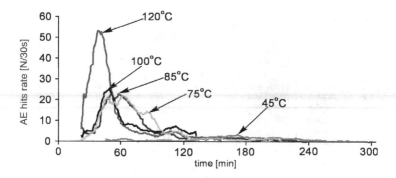

Figure 9. The rate of AE hits during drying at different temperatures

Note that the highest peak of the AE hits, which correspond to temperature 120°C, appears earlier than the lower peaks corresponding to the lower drying temperatures. The primary peak of AE hits appeared in 50 min of drying time, that is, when the tensional stresses at the cylinder surface reached maximum. The secondary peak is visible about 110 min drying time for temperature 120°C. In this time the core of the body starts to dry. The wet core wants to shrink but the surface layer is not able to deform itself because it is almost dry. So, in these circumstances the tensional stresses arise in a core. The secondary maximum is, of course, much lower than the first one.

Another AE descriptor termed *the total energy* is useful in analysis of fracture phenomenon by drying. It measures successively the total energy released during the whole process of drying. Figure 10 presents the rate of AE hits and the curve of total energy versus time.

The curve of summarized in time acoustic energy released during drying can deliver essential information on fracture dimension occurring in the investigated body. A highly fractured material is qualified as a bad quality one. The descriptor of total energy released may serve as an indicator, whether the dried product is of good or bad quality at the end-state. Strong cracks of body structure release high energetic EA signals. The high or medium energetic signals are evidenced in figure 10 as the strait upright lines. In some cases, the high energetic signals denote macro-cracks or splits that are visible on the sample surface. Taking into considerations the above presented curve of total energy one can state that it represents a dried product of bad quality.

The strength of material with damaged structure is impaired. Often a number of internal small micro-cracks arising during drying may nucleate and create macro-cracks during utilization

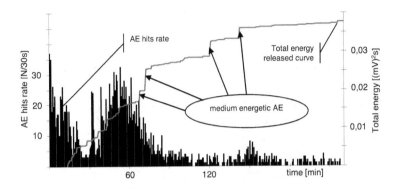

Figure 10. Total energy of AE signals released during drying

of dry products, so that an unpredictable total damage of the body may take place in any time after drying.

The reason for fracture of materials under drying results mostly from not proper drying conditions (e.g. too high temperature or too low drying medium humidity). By optimal drying process the high energetic AE signals ought to be eliminated or minimized. The majority of registered AE signals ought to be low energetic (horizontal or almost horizontal lines in figure 10). Low energetic AE signals mean lack of destruction in dried products.

Figure 11 shows several curves of total EA energy released from kaolin cylinders during drying at different temperatures. Each EA signal carries a certain portion of energy. The flat horizontal lines represent the low energetic signals. Hits of high energy create sudden vertical lines as, for example, those visible on the energy curves obtained for drying at temperatures 100 and 120°C. These very energetic signals are generated by strong material cracks.

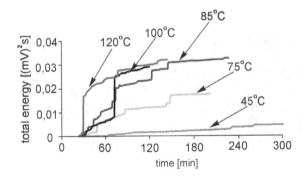

Figure 11. Total energy of hits during drying process for various conditions

Analysing figure 11 one can see the differences in released energy for different drying conditions. The curve of 45 °C, being almost horizontal, represents low energetic AE signals. It means that drying at this temperature is unpropitious for creation of material fracture, so the manufactured product is of good quality and without residual stresses. Unfortunately, drying at such a low temperature takes a long time and is unsatisfactory from the economic point of view.

The total energy curve for drying at 75°C looks a little different from that of 45°C. It contains a greater number of signals in the time period from 40 to 100 min but these signals are not so much energetic either, some of them might be generated by invisible micro-cracks. This curve is slightly inclined upwards.

The next curve (85°C) has similar character as that of 75°C one, however, represents more energetic signals. The energy released here is much higher than that represented by the two previous curves. The dried product at this temperature may have a number of micro-cracks that can expand into visible cracks under the action of residual stresses.

The most energetic AE signals are represented by the curves characterizing severe drying conditions (100°C and 120°C). So, high temperatures together with low humidity of the drying medium (air) are propitious to high drying rate. This produces quickly dry and brittle surface layers while the wet core becomes still wet and deformable. The drying induced stresses cause damage of the fragile surface.

5.2. Microwave drying of ceramic-like materials

Figure 12 presents the photographs of the cylindrical samples after microwave drying with 300 W of the microwave power (MWP). The damage of the cylinder is occurred in its center and looks like an explosion caused by a high vapor pressure inside the cylinder due to intensive phase transitions of water into vapor. This proofs that by microwave heating the highest temperature arises inside the material. It is confirmed by the picture presented in figure 12c made with infrared (IR) camera (Flir therma-cam B2).

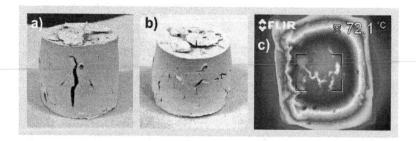

Figure 12. Kaolin sample subjected to 300 W MWP a) front view, b) rear view, c) IR camera picture of temperature distribution in the sample longitudinal cross-section

The sample subjected to 300 W of MWP has a huge vertical slit, almost 3 cm long and 2.5 cm deep (Fig. 12a). It was caused by the explosion after 20 min of drying time. The barrel shape of the samples is very clearly visible in both figures 12a and 12b. The picture of temperature distribution in the sample longitudinal cross-section (Fig. 12c) shows that the temperature reached about 90°C in some hot spots, although the mean temperature in the central part was about 72°C. This indicates the existence of places where the water was rapidly changed into vapor. The rapidly increased vapor pressure created the big slit, so that the water vapor had found the way out.

Figure 13 presents AE signals acquired during microwave drying of kaolin cylinders.

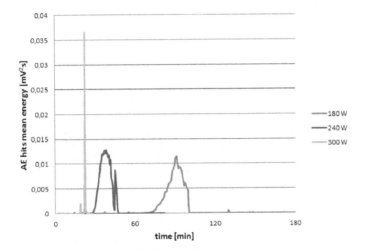

Figure 13. AE hits mean energy acquired during microwave drying of kaolin cylinders

For 300W of MWP the huge acoustic energy wave was generated during the explosion. It is visible in figure 13 as a high single signal at 20 minutes of drying. Drying with lower MWP (180 W and 240 W) induces signals of lower AE energy.

The number of AE signals induced during microwave drying depends on the MWP (Fig. 14). By lower MWP the number of AE signals is greater, but they are of lower energy than those of higher MWP.

The destruction of samples raised by microwave drying proceeds mainly in the second drying rate stage, except the one dried in 300W MWP. For samples dried in 180 W and 240W MWP-s the destruction was observed as step by step splitting small parts (Fig. 15).

The convective and microwave drying methods differ from each other in the way of heat supply. By convective drying the heat is delivered from the surroundings through the material surface from the hot air of temperature higher than the temperature of drying material. By microwave drying on the other hand the heat is generated volumetrically as a result of the

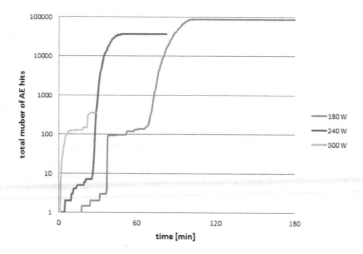

Figure 14. AE results for microwave drying of kaolin: the total number of AE hits

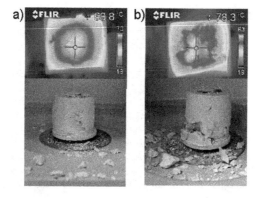

Figure 15. The kaolin sample dried in microwave oven by 240 W MWP

dispersion of the high-frequency monochrome waves of the order 2.45 GHz. The microwave power is absorbed mainly by the water present in the material pores.

The different ways of heat supply affects the directions of heat and mass fluxes. During the convective drying the heat flux is in opposite direction to the mass flux, and this causes a decrease of moisture removal, what is favorable to non-uniform distribution of the moisture inside the material. Such a negative thermodiffusive effect not appears or is minimal in microwave drying by which the heat flux coincides with the mass flux. The interior of the material usually has the temperature higher than the surroundings. The moisture distribution

in the material in this case is more uniform than during the convective drying. So the drying induced stresses should be smaller. Diagrams get from measurements of total numbers of AE signals and the AE energy confirm this prediction.

Figure 16 presents the AE hits in kaolin sample dried convectively. It appears from the presented diagrams that the maximum number of AE signals was occurred in the middle of the constant drying rate period (CDRP).

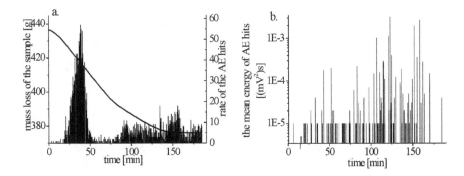

Figure 16. The AE hits for convective drying of kaolin sample: a) drying curve and AE hits rate, b) mean energy of AE hits

Kaolin clay sustains the greatest shrinkage in the initial period of drying (15 – 90 min). External layers of the cylindrical sample are dried first and shrink generating stresses and cracks, which is manifested by an increased number of AE signals. The density of these signals decreases with the course of drying, however, their energy becomes more and more greater. Figures 16a presents the rate of AE hits and 16b the mean energy of AE hits. One can see that the initial great number of hits is of relatively low energy but the subsequent ones revealed much bigger

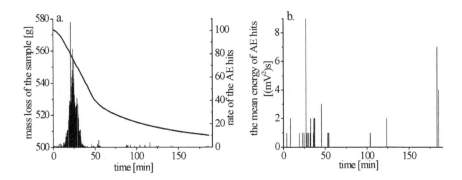

Figure 17. The AE hits by microwave drying of kaolin sample: a) drying curve and AE hits rate, b) mean energy of AE hits

energy. In the latter cases a number of distinct scratches was visible on the surface of dried samples and in some cases even micro and macro cracks were formed, particularly by drying in more severe drying conditions.

Figure 17 presents the AE hits in a kaolin sample that occurred by microwave drying. In the case of microwave drying one can see that both the number of AE hits (Fig. 17a) and the emitted AE energy (Fig. 17b) are much lower in comparison to the convective drying. The lower number of AE hits in microwave drying can be justified by the coincidence of the heat and mass fluxes and thus more uniform distribution of the moisture through the material in this kind of drying, which consequently resulted in reduction of stresses. It is important that a significant increase of drying rate was noticed by microwave drying. The CDRP amounted only from 10 to 70 min (Fig. 17a), dependent on MWP.

5.3. Convective drying of wood

Drying of pine wood samples was conducted at three different temperatures: 60, 80 and 100°C. Figure 18 presents the rate of AE hits, i.e. the density of AE signals per a time interval (e.g. 30 s) (Fig. 18a), and the drying curves (Fig. 18b), for different drying temperatures.

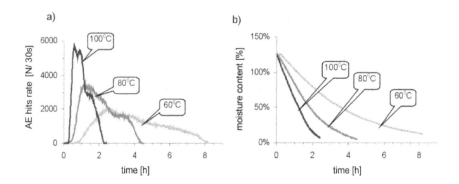

Figure 18. Results of pine wood drying: a) the rate of AE hits, b) drying curves

One can state based on the experimental results that the rate of AE hits in drying wood depends on the number and size of fractures occurred in wood samples. The shrinkage of wood begins at the moment, when the MC reaches the fiber saturation point (FSP) (c.a. 30%). In the initial drying period, when the MC in wood is higher than FSP, the AE activity is insignificant. Only when MC in the surface layers drops below FSP, and the MC inside the samples exceeds this value, the AE start to reveal greater activity, in particular for high drying temperatures. The considerable increase of the rate of AE hits corresponds then with drying temperatures and is attested by drying stresses and cracks of different sizes, which generate acoustic wave.

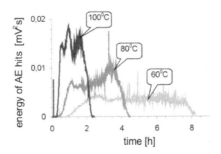

Figure 19. The energy of AE hits for pine wood sample dried at various temperatures

Figure 19 shows the energy of AE hits for pine wood for different drying temperatures. The graphs presented in this figure, and in particular this referring to drying at temperature 100°C, point out a danger of wood destruction at the moment when the AE energy reaches maximum.

As the plots in figure 19 show, the rate of AE hits grow rapidly at the beginning but after some time they decrease also quite rapidly. The rate of AE hits decreases in the period that refers to drying of the sample core, however, the emitted AE energy stays on the same level or even grows, as it is seen on the graph for 80°C. Incurred earlier micro-cracks start expanding and linking. A danger of wood destruction could be then even greater than in the initial period, because of increase of the summarized energy of AE signals. Dried wood becomes more and more rigid and the risk of the brittle cracking becomes more and more probable. Observation of the mean energy of AE hits presented in figure 20 confirms it.

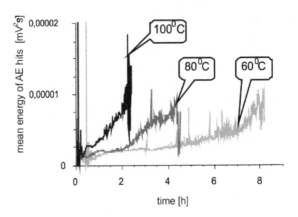

Figure 20. The mean energy of AE hits

The energy is released up to the end of drying process. Incurred earlier micro-cracks grow further. The mean energy of the AE hits is a measure of the progressing decomposition of wood. It is bigger for higher temperatures of the drying medium. However, in the conducted series of drying tests in no case occurred a visible crack of dried sample. This fact is evidenced on the curves of total energy presented in figure 21, that is, the energy summed up during the whole course of drying.

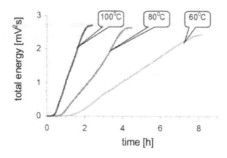

Figure 21. The total energy of AE hits for the whole drying process

One can see that the curves of total energy are growing smoothly, that is, without violent jumps. Violent jumps on graphs of total energy indicate just fractures visible even with a naked eye.

5.4. The phenomenon of stress reverse

The phenomenon of stress reverse results from a constrained shrinkage in dried material. It can happen when the surface of material becomes deformed permanently due to intensive shrinkage. The stresses arose on the surface are tensional and in the material interior compressive ones. When the drying is progressing deeper into the material and its core starts to shrink but is hindered by the surface shell previously stretched in a permanent way, then the stress on the surface becomes compressive and that in the material interior tensional, so thus the stress reverse take place.

Modeling of the stress reverse phenomenon requires taking into account inelastic properties of the materials. This issue was already considered in the work by [Kowalski, 2001, 2002; Banaszak and Kowalski, 2002; Kowalski and Rajewska, 2002; Kowalski et al., 2002].

Figure 22 shows the time evolution of the circumferential stresses distributed in the cylindrical kaolin sample dried convectively by the assumption that kaolin is viscoelastic and obey Maxwell model [Kowalski, 2001, 2002; Kowalski and Rajewska, 2002].

We can see that the circumferential stresses are compressive in the core and tensional in the boundary layer at the beginning and reversibly signed at the end of the drying process. We suppose that the tensional stresses in the core of the cylinder may cause structural fracture and thus the emission of the third group of acoustic signals at the final stage of drying.

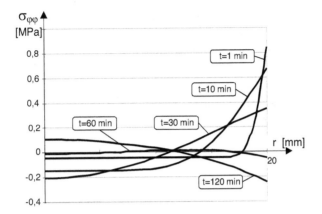

Figure 22. The evolution of circumferential stresses in kaolin cylinder dried convectively

Figure 23 shows the evolution of circumferential stresses in wooden cylinder (birch) dried convectively [Kowalski et al., 2002]. Here the Maxwell model was used for wood.

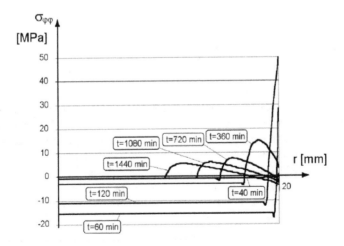

Figure 23. The evolution of circumferential stresses in wood cylinder dried convectively

At the first stage of drying the stresses for the viscoelstic model run in a similar way as for the elastic model. After some time, however, when the dry zone extends deeper towards the wet core, the circumferential stresses start to change their sign at the boundary from tensional to compressive. Note that the maximum value of the tensional circumferential stresses is moving during drying from the boundary surface towards the interior of the cylinder.

Figure 24 shows the evolution of the number of AE hits in time during convective drying of kaolin sample. The plot of the number of AE hits is confronted with the curves presented the circumferential stresses determined on the basis of elastic Hooke model (dashed line) and viscoelastic Maxwell (solid line).

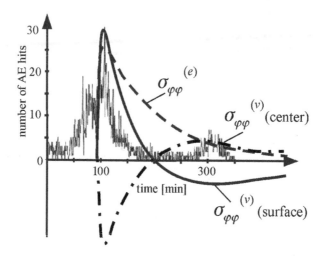

Figure 24. Hits rate and the theoretical curve of circumferential stresses as a function of time

As it is seen from figure 24, Hooke model does not reflect the occurrence of stress reverse. It demonstrates only the compliance of the first maximum of stresses with the increased AE activity. The consideration allow us to appreciate the meaning of the mathematical model adequacy for the description of the mechanical phenomena by drying of wet materials. The experimentally observed enhanced emission of acoustic signals, betoken the enhanced destruction of the material at the final stage of drying. Using the elastic model one obtains the stress development, which rises from the beginning, then reaches a maximum at point in time, and next, as the process proceeds further, disappears totally. Otherwise, the model that takes into account the permanent deformations of the dried material, allows us as in the case of viscoelastic model to observe the stress reverse, and in particular the appearance of tensional stresses inside the dried material at the final stage of drying. The tensional stresses in the core at the final stage of drying cause an increase of AE signals, which is visible in figure 24.

6. Control of material damage with the help of AE

6.1. Avoiding material fractures through changes drying conditions

The non-stationary (intermittent) convective drying denotes drying with different drying rates in several periods. The results of the drying studies presented in this chapter allows to state that the intermittent drying can be recommended above all to drying of materials, which have a tendency to cracking during drying as, for example, ceramics and wood. Through changes of drying conditions in the right moments one can avoid material fracture and thus preserve a good quality of dried products. Thus, one can state that intermittent drying positively influences the quality of the dried materials without significant extension of the drying time.

In these considerations the intermittent drying was realized through periodically changing both temperature and humidity of drying air. The results of intermittent drying are compared with adequate processes of stationary drying to show the profits resulting from the former.

Apart from the visual assessment of the quality of dried products, the acoustic emission (AE) method was applied for monitoring of the micro- and macro- cracks developed during drying [Kowalski and Pawłowski, 2010]. In those studies it was measured the total number of AE hits and the total amount of AE energy emitted. The descriptor of total AE energy is the sum of energy of all acoustic signals emitted by the dried sample from the beginning to the end of drying. It denotes the energy released due to material cracking. These descriptors show the moment at which the AE becomes intensive and how big is the AE intensity. Knowing these descriptors, one can assess the intensity of micro- and macro- cracks that arise in dried materials as well as their magnitude. The "intensity" quantifies the number of cracks per 30 s intervals or the total number of cracks in the whole process. The crack "magnitude" is evidenced as the vertical straight line on the descriptor of total AE energy curve. In this way we can estimate the degree of destruction and how fast the destruction advances in dried materials.

Figure 25 presents the total number of AE hits and the total AE energy emitted during stationary drying of the kaolin cylindrical sample at temperature 100 °C.

The plots in figure 25 show a continuous increase of the number of AE hits and the AE energy. The flatness on the energy plot that begins at about 100 min of drying follows from the release of the elastic energy accumulated in the stressed material due to material fracture, and in this way a reduction of the stress state occurs.

Figure 26 presents the total number of AE hits and the total AE energy emitted from the cylindrical sample during drying with periodically changing temperature between 50 and 100 °C in the falling drying rate period (FDRP).

Note that the total number of AE hits and the total AE energy emitted during drying with periodically changing temperature is less than those in stationary drying. The plots in figure 26 are not so smooth as those in figure 25, which follows from the variable air temperature, and strictly, by switching off and on the air heater and cooler.

Figure 27 presents the total number of AE hits and the total AE energy emitted during drying with variable air humidity. The number of emitted AE hits and the total AE energy in this kind

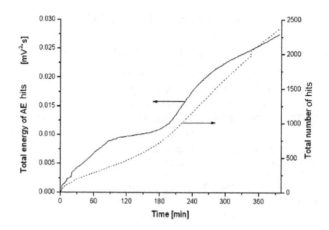

Figure 25. Total number of AE hits and total AE energy in stationary drying of cylindrical kaolin sample at 100°C

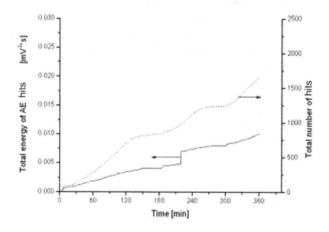

Figure 26. Total number of AE hits and total AE energy by convective drying of kaolin cylindrical sample at periodically changing temperature between 50 °C and 100 °C

of drying is lesser than those during stationary drying and also lesser than during drying with variable temperature.

The humidification of air in the chamber dryer caused the plots of acoustic emission to be very rugged. Nevertheless, we can state that drying in intermittent conditions accomplished through periodically changing temperature and air humidity is accompanied by a smaller number of AE signals and smaller value of AE energy. This denotes less micro- and macro-cracks in dried material and simultaneously better quality of dried products.

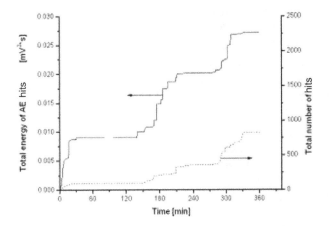

Figure 27. Total number of AE hits and total AE energy by convective drying of kaolin cylindrical sample at periodically changing air humidity between 4 % and 60 ÷ 80 %

6.2. Reduction of material fractures through surfactant application

In order to improve moisture transport inside the dried body, and thus to assure more uniform distribution of moisture in the material and thus avoid its cracking, the authors proposed wetting the raw kaolin-clay with water containing surface active agents (surfactants). These agents have the ability to stimulate the surface tension between water and the pore walls and thus to improve moisture transport inside the material [Cottrell, 1970; Wert & Thomson, 1974].

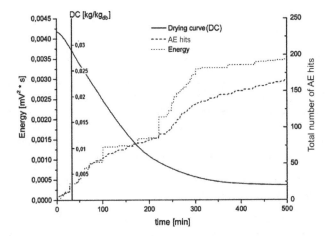

Figure 28. Drying curve, total AE energy and total number of AE hits in clay samples saturated with pure water of clay samples at air temperature 120 °C

Figure 28 presents the typical drying curve of clay samples with the CDRP (0 – 180 min) and the FDRP (180 – 400 min), and the descriptors of total AE energy and total number of AE signals emitted during drying of clay saturated with pure water.

Each rapid increase of the total AE energy visible on the AE curve denotes a crack occurring of in the clay sample at a given moment. As seen in this figure, the biggest cracks were formed in the second stage of the CDRP and in the first stage of FDRP. At this stage the sample surface became dry while the core of the sample was still wet, and material cracks occurred at this stage.

Figure 29 presents comparison of total AE energy for dried clay saturated with water containing different concentration of surfactant SDS (0, 0.001, 0.01, 0.1 and 1%).

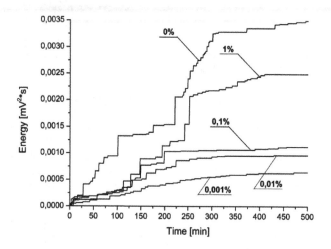

Figure 29. Comparison of total AE energy emitted by clay with different concentration of SDS

It is seen that different amounts of SDS added to water solutions used for clay saturation differentiate the total AE energy emitted by kaolin-clay during drying. As it follows from this figure, the greatest energy is emitted for clay saturated with pure water (0% SDS) and for the greatest surfactant concentration (1% SDS). It means that there is a SDS concentration at which the AE energy reaches minimum. The limit value of the surfactant concentration, at which the drying results are efficient is called *the critical micelle concentration* (CMC).

Figure 30 shows that the quality of sample with 0.01% surfactant concentration is much better than that with 0% (pure water) concentration.

Figure 30 proves that surfactant concentration of value close the CMC have a meaningful influence on moisture transport inside capillary-porous materials. These conclusion is confirmed by the good quality of dried product visualized on the photo of samples bottom surface presented in figure 30b.

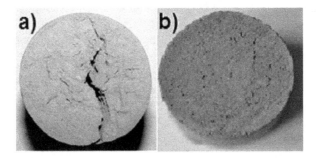

Figure 30. Bottom surface of kaolin-clay samples after drying: a) without surfactant, b) with 0.01% of SDS

7. Conclusions

The presented in this chapter results of research concerning analysis of the AE activity in dried materials allows to state that the AE method can indeed support the control of the drying process and facilitate the guidance for the purpose of avoiding destruction of materials during drying. Comparison of the drying induce stresses simulated numerically on the basis of mechanistic drying model with the experimentally measured descriptors of AE activity reveal an excellent adherence of the theoretical and experimental results. Although with the AE method we are not able to estimate strictly the magnitude of generated stresses, however, the assessment of material destruction intensity caused by the stresses and the time and place of their occurrence is very helpful for control of drying processes. Besides, monitoring of the AE events can be helpful also for validation of the failure criterion formulated on the basis of the mechanistic theory of drying, which is used for estimation of the magnitude and location of maximal stresses as well as their time evolution during drying.

It is worth to point out here the importance of the acoustic emission method that allows us observations *on line* the development of the acoustic signals connected with the destruction of the materials. The possibility of the registration of various descriptors such as: the intensity of acoustic signals, the energy of emitted signals and the total number of signals or total amount of energy allows the current control of drying processes.

Acknowledgements

This work was carried out as a part of research project No. N N209 031638 and N N209 104337 sponsored by the Polish Ministry of Education and Science.

Author details

Stefan Jan Kowalski*, Jacek Banaszak and Kinga Rajewska

*Address all correspondence to: stefan.j.kowalski@put.poznan.pl

Poznań University of Technology, Institute of Technology and Chemical Engineering, Department of Process Engineering, Poznań, Poland

References

[1] Berlinsky, Y. M, Rosen, J, & Simmons, J. Wadley HNG, ((1990). A Calibration Approach to Acoustic Emission Energy Measurement, Journal of Nondestructive Evaluation, 10 (1).

[2] Banaszak, J, & Kowalski, S. J. (2002). Drying induced stresses estimated on the base of elastic and viscoelastic models. Chem Eng J , 86, 139-143.

[3] Banaszak, J, & Kowalski, S. J. (2010). Acoustic methods in Engineering Applications, Publisher: Poznań University of Technology, Poznań (in Polish).

[4] Banaszak, J, & Kowalski, S. J. (2005). Theoretical and experimental analysis of stresses and fractures in clay like materials during drying, Chem. Engineering and Processing, , 44, 497-503.

[5] Cottrell, A. H. (1970). The mechanical properties of matter. Warsaw: PWN (in Polish).

[6] Kowalski, S. J. (2002). Theoretical study of stress reversal phenomena in drying of porous media. Dev. Chem. Eng. Mineral Process., 10(3/4): 261-280.

[7] Kowalski, S. J. (2003). Thermomechanics of Drying Processes, Springer, Berlin, Heidelberg.

[8] Kowalski, S. J. (2010). Control of mechanical processes in drying. Theory and Experiment, Chemical Engineering Science, , 65, 890-899.

[9] Kowalski, S. J, Banaszak, J, & Rybicki, A. (2012). Damage Analysis of Microwave-Dried Materials, AIChE Journal.

[10] Kowalski, S. J, & Musielak, G. (1999). Deformations and stresses in dried wood. Transport in Porous Media , 34, 239-248.

[11] Kowalski, S. J, Molinski, W, & Musielak, G. (2004). Identification of fracture in dried wood based on theoretical modeling and acoustic emission. Wood Sci Techn , 38, 35-52.

[12] Kowalski, S. J, & Pawlowski, A. (2010). Drying of wet materials in intermittent conditions,, Drying Technol. 28 (5). , 636-643.

[13] Kowalski, S. J, & Rajewska, K. (2002). Dried induced stresses in elastic and viscoelastic saturated materials. Chem Eng Sci , 57, 3883-3892.

[14] Kowalski, S. J, Rajewska, K, & Rybicki, A. (2000). Destruction of wet materials by drying, Chem. Eng. Sci. , 55, 6755-6762.

[15] Kowalski, S. J, & Rybicki, A. (1996). Drying stress formation induced by inhomogeneous moisture and temperature distribution. Transport in Porous Media , 24, 139-156.

[16] Kowalski, S. J, & Rybicki, A. (2007). The vapour-liquid interface and stresses in dried bodies, Transport in Porous Media , 66, 43-58.

[17] Luong Phong M(1994). Centrifuge simulation of Rayleigh waves in soils using a drop-ball arrangement, ASTM Special Technical Publication, (1213), 385-399.

[18] Malecki, I, & Ranachowski, J. (1994). Acoustic emission: Sources, Methods Applications, Pascal Publications, Warszawa (in Polish).

[19] Mujumdar, A. S. Ed.) ((2007). Handbook of Industrial Drying (Third Edition), Taylor & Francis Group, New York.

[20] Strumiłło Cz(1983). Fundamentals of the Theory and the Technology of Drying, WNT Warszawa, (in Polish).

[21] Wert, C. A, & Thomson, R. M. (1974). Physics of solids, National Scientific Publishers, London, UK

Structural Ageing of a Cable-Stayed Bridge During Load-Test: The Overall Effect Monitored by Acoustic Emission

Giovanni P. Gregori, Giuliano Ventrice,
Sebastiano Pinori, Genesio Alessandrini and
Francesco Bianchi

Additional information is available at the end of the chapter

1. Introduction

A study is here presented, which was carried out on a steel bridge monitored by acoustic emission (AE), during load-test before its opening to public. Other standard security checks of linear deformation were simultaneously carried out, according to law requirements, by laser monitoring.

The focus of the present study is on material fatigue, consequent to load test. This newly constructed viaduct displayed an excellent performance. Hence, it is an effective and suitable reference to be compared with every old metal viaduct. In some respect, and up to some extent, this study also applies to concrete, or brick, or wood bridges. Indeed, fatigue is a permanently ongoing process and, when integrated over time, it affects old structures, causing progressive ageing and loss of performance and security. The difference between bridges constructed by different materials only relies on a different response-time to an applied tress. But fatigue and ageing are a much similar process when dealing with different materials. There is only need for a suitable calibration focused on every given case history.

The technique here applied relies on passive AE monitoring in the ultrasound band. AE are spontaneously released by every stressed solid material. Indeed, AE occur as a response to every gentle stress, independent of its cause.

It should be pointed out that AE intensity is not of concern for the analysis which is here considered. The only requirement is that an AE signal is detectable. The timing of the AE release, not the intensity, is rather fundamental for the present analysis.

Several applications of ultrasound monitoring are reported as a standard in the literature and they deal with several engineering concerns. However, the method, which is here applied for data handling, for analysis and for physical interpretation, derives from an original procedure[1] which is completely different compared to all previous procedures by other authors that are reported in the literature.

The viaduct of the present study is named "Cavalcaferrovia Ostiense" (i.e. "Overpass Ostiense"). It holds three-lanes (altogether *11.5 m* wide) in each direction, plus two large sidewalks. It connects the major road "Circonvallazione Ostiense", on its eastern side, with the arterial road "Ostiense" on its western side (figure 1). It is ~ *159 m* long, and is located in the Rome neighbourhood named Garbatella. Hence, it is here briefly called "Garbatella bridge" (figure 2, 3 and 4).[2] Its design reminds about a 3-leg spider, with one "leg" on its eastern side. "Side A" is its northern side and "side B" its southern side. Each side is further distinguished, respectively, into its eastern (E) and western (W) segment (figures 3 and 4).

It crosses over a four-way railway, i.e. two ways of the Rome urban metro plus two ways of the suburban train Roma-Lido di Ostia. The height of the viaduct with respect to the railway[3] is comparable to the height of a train inside a standard railway tunnel. Every urban train always stops at the Garbatella station, which is very close to the viaduct (figure 1), while every suburban train crosses through it at moderate, although sometimes low, speed.

Thermal dilatation is compensated at the two western "legs" of the bridge that can slide longitudinally, while the single eastern "leg" is fixed to its concrete basement.

AE monitoring was implemented on *December 16th, 2011* on the occasion of the load test,[4] which was formally carried out on *December 17th, 2011.*[5] The total load was made by means of *28* mobile concrete mixers, filled with rubble, everyone of total weight of ~ 3.5 tons. Altogether the load was 9800 kN.

The load test was exploited in four steps. During *Step 1* the load was symmetric (*14* mixers on each side A and B). *Step 2* was asymmetric with *14* mixers on side A and no mixer on side B. *Step 3* was carried out with *5* mixers over segment A-E and *5* mixers over segment B-W. *Step 4* had a load of *8* mixers over segment A-E and *8* mixers over segment B-E.

Standard monitoring was exploited by means of laser measurements concerning several linear deformations to be compared with model computation. In addition, model computations also

---

1 The algorithms that are here applied include a few methods that already appeared in a few papers by the authors and co-workers (see below). These procedures are now also a part of a more systematic and compact set of methods for technological applications, which were implemented and patented by G. P. Gregori. Their practical exploitation and applications are in progress at S.M.E.

2 The design is by "Solidus srl – Ing. Francesco Del Tosto", with components provided by "Cimolai spa",Pordenone, Italy.

3 The road level with respect to the highest side of the rail is 7.80 m. We acknowledge and thank Ing. Francesco del Tosto for providing us with this (and other) information.

4 We acknowledge Ing. Fabio Rocchi for kindly providing with the official documentation.

5 The legal prescriptions are specified by the Italian Ministerial Decree D.M. LL. PP. 14/01/2008, Technical standards for construction, and by its explanatory supplement 02/02/2009, n. 617, Instructions for the application of the "Technical standards for construction" (D.M. 14 January 2008).

specify the axial stress of several different components of the bridge, which were compared with direct measurements.

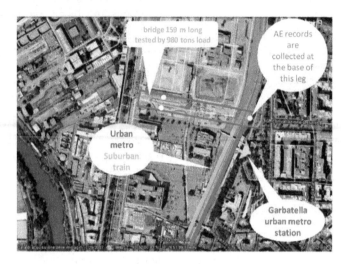

Figure 1. Sketch (out of scale), over a Google-Earth's image, showing the location of the Garbatella bridge. The urban metro line is indicated by a red strip, and the suburban train by a blue strip. The approximate locations of the three "legs" are indicated by white circles.

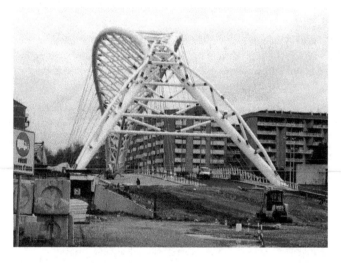

Figure 2. The Garbatella bridge seen from its western side. AE monitoring was carried out at the base of the single eastern "leg" here shown in the background.

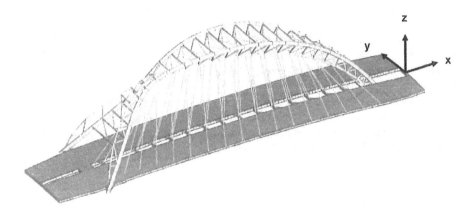

Figure 3. The 3-leg spider cable-stayed Garbatella bridge. Its single eastern leg is to the right. Figure after the official documentation of the load test of the viaduct. See text.

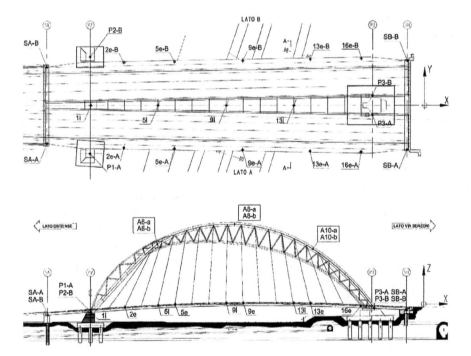

Figure 4. Horizontal and vertical orthogonal projection of the bridge. The eastern side is to the right. Figure after the official documentation of the load test of the viaduct. See text.

Only the details of *Step 1* are here of concern. The vertical displacement of the key of arch (side A) was measured as *-37 mm*, which resulted *92%* the model estimate *-40 mm*. The vertical displacement of the middle point of the road level (side A) was *59 mm*, which equals 95% the computed *62 mm*. The variation of compressive stress at the middle key of the arch (side A) resulted *-3930 kN*, which is *93%* the model estimate *-4243 kN*. The external suspension cable *9e* (side A) experienced a traction of *170 kN*, which is *97%* the estimated *175 kN*. A lower oblique chain under the road level, which opposes the longitudinal and lateral extension of the arch, experienced a traction of *3160 kN*, which is *89%* the estimated *3560 kN*. The sliding of the two western legs was (Δx, Δy, Δz, respectively, in *mm*): for the southern leg *(-11,-1,0)*, to be compared with model computation *(-12,-1,0)*, and for the northern leg *(-11,0,0)*, to be compared with model computation *(-12,1,0)*.

Similar results, which however are not here reported in detail, were found concerning *Steps 2, 3* and *4* of the load test. The absolute values of all measured parameters resulted less than the estimated applied stress. They claim that this discrepancy derived from the size of the nodes of the arch, which in model computation were assumed point-like. Therefore, the model underestimated the true rigidity of the structure.

In general, the discrepancy between model and records resulted less than a few percent, which was explained by thermal dilation effects, originated by changes of air temperature. Owing to abrupt rain and hail, at the end of *Step 1* an air temperature variation had occurred ΔT = -4°C which affected only the arch of the bridge, but not its road level, as it was protected by road cover. According to model computation, it was estimated that this effect implies a lowering to the road level by *4 mm*. The discrepancy, *4 hour* later, when the absolute value of ΔT had diminished, was only *2 mm*. This result is consistent with the leading role of the thermoelastic stress, in agreement with what is clearly envisaged by the present investigation.

For future reference, the detailed load timing is here needed only concerning *Step 1*. Two trucks at a time were loaded, starting at $08^h\ 07^{min}$ *a.m.* (LT=UT+1 hour), attaining full load at $08^h\ 45^{min}$ 45^{sec}. The loading occurred by adding 3 sets of mixers at a time. The first set, here called "load-1" set, involved 7 couples of trucks loaded during *9 min* (approximately at $08^h\ 07^{min}$, $08^h\ 08^{min}$, $08^h\ 10^{min}\ 45^{sec}$, $08^h\ 12^{min}$, $08^h\ 13^{min}$, $08^h\ 15^{min}$, $08^h\ 16^{min}$ LT). Then, 2 couples of trucks were loaded after a while (approximately at $08^h\ 24^{min}$ and $08h\ 34^{min}\ 15^{sec}$); this is here denoted as "load-2" set. The remaining 6 couples of trucks were loaded during *5.5 min* (approximately at 08^h 42^{min}, $08^h\ 43^{min}$, $08^h\ 43^{min}\ 30^{sec}$, $08^h\ 45^{min}$, $08^h\ 45^{min}\ 45^{sec}$), and this is here denoted as "load-3" set.

The load test further continued through *Steps 2, 3* and *4*. But, their detailed timing is not of interest for the present study. The entire load test was completed by late afternoon.

2. AE monitoring

AE were recorded (figure 5) at the base of the single eastern "leg", in two frequency bands: high frequency (HF AE) at *200 kHz* and low frequency (LF AE) at *25 kHz*.

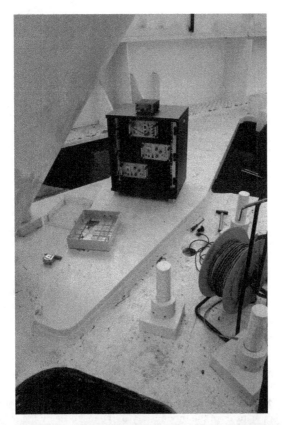

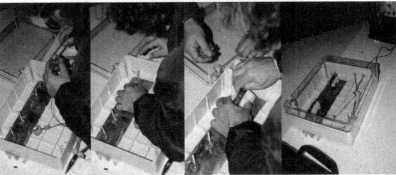

Figure 5. The AE recording apparatus while it is implemented (upper figure), and details of the AE detector (lower figure), where every AE transducer is located inside a transparent plastic cylinder (left figure), and the two preamplifiers are the small white cylinders (right figure).

Per each frequency, the primary signal was released by a piezoelectric acoustic transducer. The signal was then pre-amplified and amplified. The rms amplitude of the signal was averaged over *5 msec*. The entire set of all these [*5 msec*]-averaged signals was averaged over a pre-chosen time interval *Δt*. Then, a data logger stored this final average over *Δt* into two distinct data series, for HF AE and LF AE, respectively.

The main time series of records lasted between *Dec 16th 20h 58min 59sec* through *Dec 29th 14h 17min 35sec*. Data were collected at *Δt=4 sec* and these series are here briefly denoted as the "*4s*" data set. It is almost uninterrupted, apart a few minor gaps. During one of these gaps, between *Dec 20th 12h 14min 58sec* through *Dec 20th 13h 39min 11sec*, data were recorded with *Δt=1 sec* and these series are here briefly denoted as "*1s*" set.

Meteorological conditions were substantially perturbed, with occasional relevant wind gusts, and episodic rain or hail precipitation. However, no anemometer was available, and no regular temperature record.

3. Data analysis: Algorithms and physical principle

Data handling was carried out by a set of a few different algorithms. Reference is made to previous literature[6]. Several applications of these methods already appeared in previous papers by the authors and co-workers, mainly concerned with the natural environment (crustal stress and volcanic precursors), but including also a few studies dealing with laboratory test, either on steel or on (non-reinforced) concrete.

The present paper is specifically focused on the output of a few algorithms, which are better suited to characterize the *overall* performance of the steel structure. Additional algorithms are to be later considered by additional investigations (in preparation), to be more specifically concerned with detailed features of the time-history of the response by the microcrystalline solid structure to the applied stress, both during load-time and during after-load recovery.

The identical data handling and analysis has been separately applied to both HF AE and LF AE series.

One key algorithm, here applied and briefly summarized, deals with the fractal dimension D_t of the time series of the AE records.

But a preliminary needed step is the *outlier rejection* which is applied to every AE raw data series. The purpose is to get rid of every AE signal that, owing to any physical reason (maybe sometimes even by unpredictable instrumental bad functioning but also by any other un-wanted physical disturbance), eventually appears to deviate by a relevant amount with respect

---

6 As far as the methods are concerned, refer to Paparo et al. (2002, 2006), Gregori et al. (2002, 2005, 2007, 2012), Paparo and Gregori (2003), Gregori and Paparo (2004), and Poscolieri et al.(2006, 2006a), where several applications are discussed in detail. Other applications are here mentioned passim. Additional references dealing with applications and which are not mentioned in the following are: for laboratory experiments on concrete see Guarniere (2003) and Gregori and Paparo (2006); for Vesuvius see Paparoet al. (2004, 2004a); for Cephallonia Island see Lagios et al. (2004), and Poscolieri et al. (2006); and for fractal analysis on the geographical distribution of faults see Cello (2000) and Gregori et al. (2010).

to some "smooth" trend of its background. However, while dealing with every previous analogous AE investigation, the outlier series resulted *not* to be concerned with spurious and unwanted disturbances. Rather, it reflected an intrinsic physical feature, derived from the intimate physics of the microcrystalline structure of materials (see section 4). This same conclusion is also found in the present study.

The subsequent investigation of the outlier series, which is here reported, is then carried out by the algorithm *"arp"*, which in the present application resulted particularly suited for the detection of some (maybe unexpected) oscillations of the bridge.

The algorithm for outlier rejection relies on some mathematical technicalities, which are not of specific interest for the present discussion. Therefore, owing to brevity purposes, they are not here explained. The interested reader may refer to the aforementioned literature.

Call $f(t)$ the data series of the records (of either HF AE or LF AE). It is a discrete set of values. In general, all values refer to successive time instants defined by a time increment Δt. According to the requirements by our algorithm, however, this regularity is only optional. For the *1s* set it is $\Delta t = 1\ sec$, and for the *4s* set it is $\Delta t = 4\ sec$. Reject the outliers.

Call $\bar{f}(t)$ a (weighted) running mean, computed only by means of the *non-rejected* $f(t)$. In the present analysis, a triangular weight-function was chosen with half-time interval $\pm\ 100\ sec$. This interval, however, may be arbitrarily changed inside comparatively loose constraints, and this choice results to imply only a physically insignificant consequence on results.

Call $g(t) = f(t) - \bar{f}(t)$ the residual, computed by means of all $f(t)$, i.e. *including* also the formerly rejected outliers.

Define a point-like process[7] identified with the time series of "AE events" defined as follows.

An "AE event" is identified with *one relative maximum* of $g(t)$. But the amplitude of this relative maximum must to be above some arbitrarily pre-defined *threshold*, defined as follows.

Consider a reasonably wide subset of the original series of $g(t)$. Call "*S*" this subset. Compute the rms value σ of all $g(t)$ contained in "*S*". In the present case, the aforementioned threshold has been chosen as $[\sigma/4]$ for the reasons explained below.

Choose another arbitrary and suitable time interval Δt_1, which is used to evaluate D_t. For every given pre-chosen time instant t_j (for $j=1, 2,...$), consider the set "*M*" of all elements of the aforementioned point-like process, which occur inside a moving time lag of total duration Δt_1 and centred at the given t_j. Apply the box counting method,[8] and compute the fractal dimension $D_t(t_j)$ (for $j=1, 2,...$) of the set "*M*". This $D_t(t_j)$ is one leading parameter in the present discussion.

---

7 A "point-like process" is the conventional name used in mathematics to denote a time series of "yes" events (e.g. a heartbeat, a natural catastrophe, an earthquake of magnitude larger than a given threshold, a volcanic eruption, a flood, etc.). Every event is characterized by its abscissa (i.e. time in the present case history), independent of its ordinate (or intensity).

8 This is a well known algorithm and its description may be easily found on every elementary textbook on fractal analysis.

The criterion used for the definition of the aforementioned *threshold* began by choosing ten trial values for the threshold, everyone arbitrarily defined as $[\sigma/k]$ (with $k=1, 2,..., 10$). The fractal dimension $D_t(k)$ was computed on the entire aforementioned subset "S", and for every given k.

Owing to physical reasons, if k is exceedingly large, a threshold chosen equal to $[\sigma/k]$ results exceedingly small. The background noise is thus included and some false "AE events" enter into subsequent computation: owing to its mathematical definition, a large $D_t(k)\sim1$ must therefore be found.

In contrast, if k is exceedingly small, $[\sigma/k]$ results exceedingly large, and the threshold excludes several physically significant "AE events", which are erroneously likened to background.

Therefore, owing to mathematical reasons, the plot of $D_t(k)$ *vs.* k certainly is monotonic and decreasing. But, whenever a step-like decrease is observed on this plot, this denotes the correct k value, which excludes the entire background noise, while it keeps all values which are physically significant. Hence, this k defines the correct logical "sieve" that rejects noise and saves the physical significant information. The optimum choice was thus found to be $k=4$.

However, in the present data analysis - and concerning both *1s* and *4s* sets - it is convenient to consider the definition of Δt_1 from a different viewpoint. Let us refer to the *order number* of the elements of the point-like process, rather than to their respective *time instant*. In the present application, this makes no difference, as the original AE data series was recorded at constant time increments Δt.

Three choices have been made for each *1s* or *4s* set. Every single $D_t(t_j)$ was computed by means of N_D elements, which are included in the aforementioned Δt_1 moving time lag. It was chosen either $N_D =600$, or $N_D =1200$, or $N_D =1800$ elements. In the case of the *1s* data series, this implies that the evaluation of every $D_t(t_j)$ was carried out by referring to running time intervals of total duration *10 min, 20 min*, and *30 min*, respectively. In the case of the *4s* data series, this corresponded to evaluate a $D_t(t_j)$ by referring to time intervals of *40 min, 80 min*, and *2 hours*, respectively.

These different choices of N_D were considered, because a different N_D eventually plays a relevant role when dealing with the error-bar and scatter of the time series of computed $D_t(t_j)$ ($j=1, 2,...$). The reason is the unknown response to unwanted disturbances, originated by several physical environmental perturbations (see section 5). This N_D choice resulted comparably critical for HF AE, while concerning LF AE series it appeared robust.

As already mentioned, other algorithms for data analysis are to be considered (in preparation), which are more directly focused on details of the response of the microcrystalline steel structure. But, as far as the present analysis is concerned, only one relevant physical item ought to be here anticipated.

According to the so-called "hammer effect" (see Gregori *et al.*, 2007), we found that, in the present AE records, the AE release almost always occurs *only* during the "recovery stage", rather than during the "hammer stage". That is, no AE release occurs while the material is subjected, on an instant basis, to an externally applied stress. Rather, the AE release occurs as soon as the micro-crystals recover during their (approximately) "elastic" response, after the former applied stress. But, owing to brevity purposes, no additional details can be here given.

Another algorithm used for the present study is the "*arp*" histogram[9] applied to both outliers time series. This algorithm may be applied to every point-like process. Every event is considered independent of its intensity, and only the time instant of its occurrence is considered. Call $\{t_j\}$ $(j=1, 2,...)$ the time series of a point-like process, and call $\Delta t_{j,k}$ $(j,k= 1, 2,....; k>j)$ the set of *all* possible time intervals between the time instants of *any* couple of successive (even non-contiguous in time) elements of the set $\{t_j\}$.

"*Arp*" is the histogram of these $\Delta t_{j,k}$ $(j,k= 1, 2,....; k>j)$. But, it is well known that a histogram can be drawn only after choosing a suitable elementary time increment Δt_e on abscissas, such that all the elements that occur during every given time interval Δt_e of the histogram are supposed to be associated with an identical occurrence instant of time. Practically, it resulted convenient to define Δt_e equal to $(1/10)$ the average of all $\Delta t_{j,k}$ $(j,k= 1, 2,....; k>j)$.

As it can be easily shown (just try it), owing to definition, if the point-like process is a random series, its "*arp*" must look like a rectangular triangle, with a regularly decreasing trend. In contrast, if the system has some leading component characterized by a periodicity T_0, its "*arp*" will display approximately the same roughly decreasing trend, and a scatter superposed on it with relative maxima at every abscissa hT_0 $(h=1,2,...)$.

Denote by T any general value for an abscissa of "*arp*" abscissas and call $n(T)$ its ordinate. The error bar of "*arp*" is expressed as $n(T) \pm \sqrt{n(T)}$. Since this error bar depends on $n(T)$, the assessment may eventually result ambiguous of the occurrence of a relative maximum of $n(T)$. This drawback can, however, be easily avoided by considering the histogram defined by $\sqrt{n(T)} \pm 1/2$, which has a constant error bar, and will be here briefly denoted as $\sqrt{arp}$.

In the next section a concise summary is given of the primary physical principle. This is the basis for entire physical rationale of all previous algorithms. Section 5 deals with the analysis of D_t and with the way to recognize and rebut unwanted environmental disturbances. Section 6 deals with the "*arp*" (or $\sqrt{arp}$) analysis of each outlier series.

4. The physical rationale

No material exists that is either ideally "elastic", or ideally "plastic". Every time that every real approximately "elastic" and solid medium experiences a stress, it also experiences a fatigue. For instance, even a tenuous thermal deformation is a cause of ageing of the medium.

The fatigue, or ageing, of the material is manifested as a rupture of some crystalline bond. Whenever an additional stress is applied, new bonds yield. But, in general, these new ruptures occur close to formerly broken bonds, where the crystalline structure is comparatively weaker.

---

9 "Arp" is an acronym for "automatic research of periodicities". "Arpa" is the Italian name for harp.

In this way, a true chain-reaction occurs. This is the physical explanation of the well known phenomenon of cleavage plane in a crystal.

Every time that a crystalline bond yields, some AE is released, which is propagated through the medium. The primary physical information of our method relies on the timing of the sequence of subsequent AE release, which is detected inside the medium.

It should be pointed out that the concern is not about the intensity of the AE signal. There is only need to assume that the signal has a sufficient intensity in order that it can be detected. Indeed, the recorded AE amplitude is controlled by several unknown factors, such as by the distance and intensity of the instant AE source, but also by the unknown and eventually time-varying damping of the signal between source and detector, etc.

In contrast, the *timing* of the detected AE signal results to be an information of paramount importance in order to check how the medium responds to an applied stress. In this way, the ageing of the medium can be effectively monitored, and its eventual loss of performance. The entire procedure is therefore purely passive, and no invasive action is required.

An important related concept deals with the *frequency* of the AE signal, which depends on the size of the micro-flaw, which is associated with the broken bonds: comparatively smaller flaws release comparatively higher frequencies. We cannot know the law that relates flaw size and AE frequency, but we do know that this is the physically correct rationale.

While the ageing process is in progress, small flaws coalesce into larger ones. A former population of comparatively smaller flaws thus progressively decays, while it generates an increasing population of larger flaws etc.

Define "flaw domain" (Gregori *et al.*, 2012) the typical physical domain of a flaw, which is associated with the observed AE of a given frequency (although we do not know the real size of this flaw domain). The statistics of flaw domains for a given AE frequency shall display a lognormal distribution.

This inference derives by consideration of the rationale of the simplest case history of the so-called Kapteyn class distributions (Kapteyn, 1903, 1912; Katpeyn and van Uven, 1916; Paparo and Gregori, 2003). That is, the probability of occurrence of an event is proportional to the number of identical events that are occurring at the same instant of time. For details and reference see the aforementioned literature. Owing to definition, a lognormal distribution is asymmetric. It has a tail, and this can be promptly shown to be the primary physical cause for the aforementioned persistence of outliers, both in $f(t)$ and in $g(t)$, independent of the "sieve".

We know therefore that one and the same kind of anomalous behaviour is to be expected to be observed first by AE of comparatively higher frequency, and subsequently by AE of every progressively lower frequency, etc. This is of paramount important, as it provides us with a *physical* information on the *direction of the time arrow* inside the ageing process. That is, we can thus recognize a *precursor* phenomenon compared to an *after-event* occurrence. For instance, in the case of seismic precursors, or of any kind of other environmental measurements, the practically unsolvable problem is well known of the assessment, on a statistical basis, of what is a *precursor* compared to what is an *aftershock*.

Summarizing, it is possible to monitor the ageing of a material - and the loss of performance of a structure (either natural or manmade) - simply by a passive monitoring of the AE released by its medium, when it responds even to a very gentle stress.

When an AE experiment is carried out in the laboratory, we can very effectively control the physical system, and by this we can minimize the impact of unwanted disturbances. In contrast, when operating in the field, this is impossible, and it is therefore important to record environmental perturbations in order to assess their respective impact on the AE records and on their interpretation.

While exploiting the AE monitoring of the Garbatella bridge, unfortunately no regular meteorological records were available. Hence, the meteorological disturbances had to be assessed by means of an *a posteriori* analysis on both AE data series.

In this respect it has to be pointed out that we deal with D_t which is treated like a *performance index*. Its temporal trend is considered and, on its basis, an eventual alert is to be issued according to some pre-defined and well assessed protocol.

But, in general, while evaluating the D_t *vs. t* trend, two distinct operative case histories are thus to be envisaged.

• In one case, every AE event primarily responds to one applied stress impulse, which is originated by an external action applied to the system. For instance, consider the case history of a volcano. Its endogenous hot fluids eventually repeatedly and progressively increase their pressure. The pores of the medium of the volcanic edifice experience an ever increasing number of yielding of flaw domains. As long as the solid structure of the medium affords to sustain the increasing pressure, it is found that D_t remains reasonably small. But, when the pressure increases, also D_t shall increase, as an ever increasing number of flaw domains will randomly yield per unit time. When D_t increases until reaching 1 the volcanic edifice shall unavoidably yield, and a new boca is opened. This time sequence was observed e.g. on the occasion of the recent Stromboli paroxysm (Gregori and Paparo, 2006).

• The second case history is to be considered when the externally applied stress is only a trigger, and we observe only the subsequent evolution of the medium, while it searches for a new equilibrium state, after having suffered by the previously applied stress. In this case, a "young" medium first responds with a D_t close to 1, because the ruptures of its bonds occur randomly, as no previously organized flaw domains exist inside it. In contrast, an "aged" medium will display a progressively decreasing D_t and the lower is D_t the more "aged" is the medium.

For instance, while carrying out experiments on some steel bars (Biancolini *et al.*, 2006), it was found that when $D_t \sim 0.45$-0.5 the bar is very close to break (different steels ought, however, to be tested in the laboratory, in order to assess an eventually different security threshold for different alloys).

Differently stated, D_t denotes how far every AE event keeps a memory of other AE events either that occurred before it, or that are going to occur after it. No memory exists in a random sequence of AE event, the medium is therefore "young", and it is found D_t =1, just due to the mathematical definition of randomness. When the medium suffers by progressive ageing, its flaw domains get progressively organized towards the final organization of a cleavage plane. This entire process is illustrated and quantitatively measured by the time evolution of D_t towards progressively lower values.

5. Steel ageing — The D_t analysis, and the rejection of environmental disturbances

Concerning the AE monitoring of the Garbatella bridge, for clarity and brevity purposes let us anticipate a few much general inferences and conclusions.

A higher temporal resolution ought to be recommended. An AE datum ought to be recorded, at least, every *50-100 msec* (rather than every *1 sec* or every *4 sec*).

Consider the warning of section 4. When the external trigger caused by an environmental agent is repetitive, displaying some peculiar time sequence, the resulting AE signal - when it is interpreted according to the present rationale - may eventually simulate a false effect. Therefore, while one operates in the field, a sum of unknown and unpredictable disturbances must always be suitably taken into account, and whenever needed rejected.

This drawback is found to be particularly severe for HF AE, which are much more directly related to the primary external input. In contrast, owing to physical reasons (see section 4), the LF AE are more directly related to the downgrading of the crystalline structure. Indeed, LF AE are released when the material has already evolved and some conspicuous amount of comparatively large flaw domains have already been generated. Therefore, LF AE are to be expected to be much more indicative of the real loss of performance of a structure, while HF AE ought to be much better representative of the diachronic history of its external disturbances.

In terms of an expressive analogy, it is like listening music while a child close to you abruptly and loudly cries. The child noise has to be rebutted in order to appreciate the music in the background. Similarly, the ageing of the structures can be appreciated only after rejecting unwanted, even "loud", disturbances.

Summarizing, the primary scope of the analysis of a data series measured in the field is the distinction between the effects associated with the unknown timing of some external input, compared to the time history of the AE release determined by the evolution of the ageing process inside the medium which is to be monitored. In addition, the "perturbation" by external causes, which may eventually simulate a false behavior, is much better evidenced by means of HF AE compared to LF AE.[10]

One additional relevant concern, related to the role of the external trigger, deals with a technological problem, i.e. with the time required by the whole AE recording device to reach

---

10 This conclusion is evident from the "macro-analysis" which is here presented. But it is also confirmed by a much more detailed - "micro" rather than "macro" – analysis, which is the object of a different investigation (in preparation).

its operative regime. During a limited initial time-lag, a sum of several normally unknown factors apparently perturb the AE records. This lag has to be empirically determined, mostly whenever one wants to carry out once in a while a rapid test of performance of a given structure (the purpose is to avoid, sometimes and whenever possible, a steady AE monitoring, which is comparatively more expensive and time consuming).

Summarizing, we have to distinguish (mainly for HF AE but also in LF AE) between AE signals caused by an accidental trigger compared to the AE signals which are passively released by the material and are specifically suited to monitor its ageing.

It is therefore here first shown how we first assessed the role of a few typical and relevant disturbances. The Garbatella bridge is "young" and performing. The target of the present test-experiment is therefore to calibrate the procedure of AE analysis, in order to check and assess a general procedure suited to investigate the performance of every old bridge.

We thus realized that - compared to the time of its formal load test - the viaduct suffered by a comparatively greater stress during the previous day, when the road cover was laid down.

Figure 6 is a plot of the raw signal for both HF AE and LF AE $4s$ sets, while the $1s$ set is discussed only here below, when dealing with a specific item (see figure 22). An exponential decay trend is superposed on either plot to represent the recovery of the bridge after the stress that was applied during *Dec 16th* and *17th*. The HF AE time-constant of the decay is about half the time-constant for LF AE, consistently with the fact that HF AE, compared to LF AE, are more directly associated with a shorter-lived effect.

For future reference, it should be pointed out that the HF AE signal is very low, almost null (although not strictly null; see below) except during the warmer hours of the day (say between noon and 5 p.m.). This denotes that the signal amplification was insufficient in order to detect the AE signal other than when the thermoelastic deformation was conspicuous. This is a typical case history that shows that the instrumental amplification of the original AE signal was suitable only during some hours of the day, while during other hours the recording system was in underflow.

The most important inference which deals with material ageing is represented by $D_t(t_j)$ computed for LF AE and by the $4s$ data set (figure 7). The three different computations, by $N_D=600$, or $N_D=1200$, or $N_D=1800$ for every $D_t(t_j)$ computation, result remarkably similar.

Every apparently much dramatic very low value for $D_t(t_j)$ is the expected response to every sporadic disturbance originated by finishing works in progress on the viaduct. The viaduct was not open to public, and a conspicuous amount of finishing activity was in progress during the ~ *13 days* spanned by the $4s$ set. Drills were occasionally used, operated inside either the metal components or the concrete basement of the "legs". Since the bridge is a very efficient AE probe, composed of a monolithic body with an excellent conduction of ultra-sounds, the action of a drill - or of any kind of strong friction which causes some relevant local destruction of crystalline bons – must produce an LF AE signal with some very low $D_t(t_j)$. This is the same effect as the aforementioned "loud" disturbance by the cry of a child while you listen music.

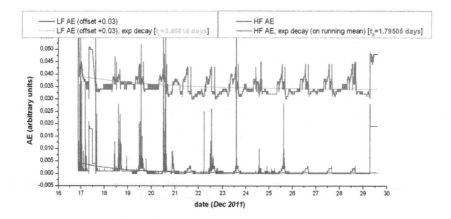

Figure 6. Raw data of the *4s* data sets. The cause is unknown of the abrupt upward discontinuity at time instant *29,28337* (it was probably instrumental while disassembling the AE recording device). An overall interpolated exponential decay is superposed (computed on $\bar{f}(t)$ for LF AE and on $f(t)$ for HF AE and by excluding the unreliable final discontinuity). The time constant is *1.795 ± 0.016 days* for HF AE and *3.468 ± 0.043 days* for LF AE. That is, the recovery of steel after load-test is about twice more rapid for HF AE compared to LF AE flaw domains. Note that the detected HF AE signal is significant only during the warmer hours of the day, while during the remaining hours in general the AE detecting system is in underflow. See text.

Another cause of much dramatic very low value for $D_t(t_j)$ is the eventual underflow of the AE detection device. Indeed, if the recorded AE signal is e.g. constant in time (e.g. at its lowest sensitivity value, i.e. *1 mV* on the scale plotted in the figures here shown), it is found $D_t(t_j)=0$. This can be formally checked, but it also represents the fact that, when all AE records are identical, the physical system has a complete memory of all AE records which occur at every other instant of time.

Note that all these features are evident independent of N_D. The algorithm is robust. The real relevant information about the ageing of the metal components of the viaduct is therefore represented by the long-range trend of the average value of $D_t(t_j)$, which is found to be intuitively close to $D_t \sim 0.8$.

The analogous D_t time series for HF AE, shown in figure 8, denotes a comparably less robust response to the N_D choice, but no clear inference. When the AE recording system is underflow (see figure 6) no D_t can be computed, according to the argument mentioned here above. Figure 8 displays therefore an approximately diurnal periodical trend, because the system detects AE signals, with a significant time-varying intensity, only during the warmer hours of the day.

Therefore, we smoothed the $D_t(t_j)$ data series by means of a weighted running average, with triangular weight over *6 min 40 sec*. The result for HF AE is shown in figure 9, which displays three time intervals with comparably much different trend. The initial and final time intervals appear to be steadily increasing. At present, it has been impossible to envisage the physical reason of this behaviour. Environmental disturbances ought to be monitored, dealing either

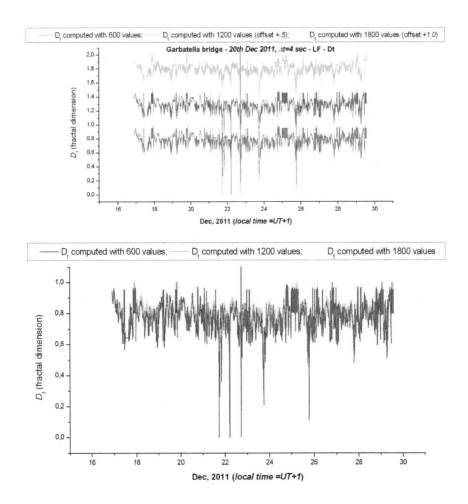

Figure 7. Fractal dimension $D_t(t_j)$ computed for LF AE of the *4s* data set, by using $N_D = 600$, or $N_D = 1200$, or $N_D = 1800$. The same values are plotted with offset (upper plot) or superposed (lower plot). The excellent performance of the viaduct is shown by the average trend at a steady $D_t(t_j) \sim 0.8$ value, while the scatter is caused by wind gusts and/or by the finishing activity that was in progress on the bridge and/or by underflow of the AE recording device. See text.

with meteorology or with manmade actions. In addition, long data series ought to be always recommended, in order to avoid boundary fringe-effects that, at least in principle, can never be fully avoided. In contrast, the intermediate time interval displays an exponential recovery, with a time constant *2.687 ± 0.066 days* which is of the same order of magnitude (*~1.8 days*) of the time constant displayed in figure 6.

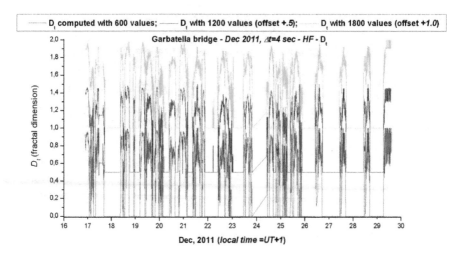

Figure 8. Fractal dimension $D_t(t_j)$ computed by HF AE of the *4s* data set. Only the plot with offset is shown. Compared to LF AE, this plot appears somewhat less robust with respect to the choice of N_D. When the AE recording system is underflow no D_t can be computed. Hence, this plot displays an apparent diurnal variation, because D_t can be computed only when AE records are available, i.e. only during the warmer hours of every day when a conspicuous thermoelastic effect was ongoing. See text.

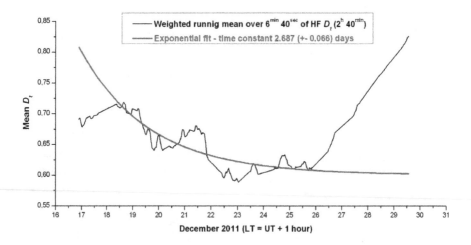

Figure 9. Weighted running average of $D_t(t_j)$ for HF AE by a triangular weight over ±3 *min 20 sec*. The initial and final steadily increasing trend is unexplained, and it is likely to be maybe associated to environmental disturbances or fringe effects. The exponential trend of the intermediate time lag displays a time constant *2.687 ± 0.066 days*, which is of the same order of magnitude of the time constant displayed in figure 6. See text.

The same procedure was applied to the LF AE data series. Figure 10 shows quite a different result. No regular exponential decay is anymore clearly detectable. Rather, the steel responds abruptly to every temporary time-varying externally applied stress. This is particularly evident on *Saturday Dec 24th*, *Sunday Dec 25th*, and *Monday Dec 26th*, because, owing to Christmas' holiday, basically no working activity was in progress on the bridge, which was rather subjected only to atmospheric disturbances.

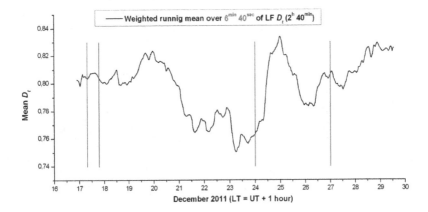

Figure 10. Weighted running average of $D_t(t_j)$ for LF AE by a triangular weight over 3 *min 20 sec.*. The load test on *Dec 17th* is evidenced by blue lines, and the holiday time on *Dec 24th*, *25th*, *26th*, by red lines. See text.

This means that HF AE, compared to LF AE, reflect a substantially much different feature of steel behaviour. HF AE reflect some much preliminary response, compared to LF AE which rather detect the substantial subsequent implications for crystalline structure, which are manifested as a later consequence of the primary applied external stress.

In any case, the prompt performance and reliability appears evident of this "young" via-duct, even during this much disturbed period of time, because the steel response denotes a rapid recovery after every applied stress, which promptly brings back the $D_t(t_j)$ value to a high and reliable level. Therefore, the medium is performing, even though the bridge, as a whole, has a slow recovery, as displayed in figure 6. In contrast, in the case of an older bridge, it is reasonable to expect that the steel ought to result much less performing, being denoted by a lower mean D_t trend.

In this respect, two laboratory tests ought to be recalled. A perfectly "young" material has an ideal abstract value $D_t(t_j)=1$. In contrast, its ageing is monitored by the relative decrease of $D_t(t_j)$. An experiment on some suspension blades of martensitic steel (Braccini *et al.*, 2002) showed a progressive decrease from $D_t(t_j) \sim 1$ (when the blade was never bent after melting) to $D_t(t_j) \sim 0.6$ (after it had been bent only a few times). Then, the crystalline structure of the martensitic steel apparently attained its working regime. Thus, it finally displayed a steady performance.

Only after some heavy and repeatedly applied stress, a steel bar is to be expected to break. Experiments carried out on small steel bars (Biancolini *et al.*, 2006) were pushed until final rupture of every specimen. It was thus found that that when it is $D_t(t_j) \sim 0.45 - 0.5$ the steel is almost close to total rupture. It should be stressed, however, that these alert values ought to be calibrated for every specific steel alloy.

Hence, it has to be expected that, in the future, the $D_t(t_j)$ of the Garbatella bridge ought to decrease until reaching a standard and steady working regime [maybe $D_t(t_j) \sim 0.6$ if the same threshold applies for the steel of the viaduct compared to the steel of the aforementioned laboratory experiment on martensitic blades]. This $D_t(t_j) \sim 0.6$ will characterize its perform-ance during the largest part of its existence. In contrast an old bridge, with collapse hazard, ought to have already slowly approached its final alert threshold of $D_t(t_j)$. It should be al-ways stressed, however, that this threshold has to be assessed, in every case history, upon considering the specific kind of steel by which it was constructed.

As far as the cause of the scatter is concerned of raw data and of $D_t(t_j)$, no anemometer re-cords were available. Hence, the role of wind can be only indirectly investigated in the present study. During those days strong gusts of wind frequently occurred. According to the personal witness of the two co-authors (SP and GV) who set up and operated the instru-ments, on the occasion of every wind gust the recording device experienced strong transient perturbations, mostly in HF AE. Hence, they tuned the signal amplification on these wind gusts, and the HF AE recording device later resulted in underflow during calm periods, with low thermal excursion.

In any case, as far as the available AE data are concerned, several different specific kinds of disturbances can be distinguished and recognized as explained in the following subsections.

5.1. Thermoelasticity, and the effect of a time-varying load

Figure 11 is a superposed epoch representation of LF AE records of the *4s* set. The smoothed function $\overline{f}(t)$ is superposed, instead of the raw data, in order to reduce scatter. A few physical facts are clearly evidenced, and a few days are indicated by a label on the figure.

During the entire *Dec 16th* heavy works were in progress on the viaduct, when a thick first layer of material was posed on the bridge for roadbed preparation. According to an indicative estimate, a *6 cm* layer of binder was laid down, with a total load of $\sim 200 \text{ tons}$ on each 3-lane way. In addition, construction machines were used, which had a total weight of $\sim 100 \text{ tons}$.[11]

After *9 p.m.* of *Dec 16th* until *7 a.m.* of the *Dec 17th*, the bridge was recovering after its violent stress.

During *Dec 17th* (red line), at ~8 a.m., the load-test was started, with dramatic consequences on the LF AE signal. Note that the straight line is associated with a period of time during which no records were available, due to a temporary failure of power supply.

---

11 We thank Ing. Francesco Del Tosto for providing us with this information.

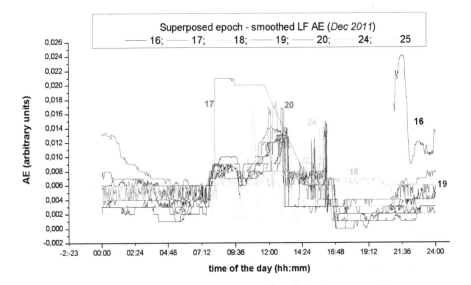

Figure 11. Superposed epoch representation (or "cycle diagram" for *24 hour* period) of the LF AE records of the *4s* set. The smoothed function $\tilde{f}(t)$ is used instead of raw data in order to reduce the scatter. The labels on a few colored lines are the date (*Dec 2011*). No offset was applied. The difference between the lowest level of different days day depends on the relaxation process shown in figure 6. Note the dramatic behavior during the late *Dec 16th* and early *Dec 17th* consequent to the stress applied while laying down the roadbed. See text.

During the subsequent days, the most intense LF AE signal was recorded during working hours (say roughly between *8 a.m.* through *5 p.m.*), envisaging an effects associated with the stress applied while finishing the bridge.

But, it appears curious the fact that also on *Dec 25th*, Christmas Day, when no work was ongoing on the bridge (yellow line), some relevant LF AE signal was observed. In addition, in general, on every day a comparatively more intense signal was recorded almost at the same local time, i.e. during the early afternoon until ~ *4 p.m.* Therefore, this appears to be a likely thermoelastic effect.

In addition, in general a reasonably ordered and regular scatter was observed every day before *7 a.m.* (except on *Dec 17th*, when the bridge was recovering after the stress of the previous day). In contrast, the comparative trend on different days after *6 p.m.* appears more varied, maybe depending on different air temperature (for which, however, no record is available).

All these features are suggestive of a thermoelastic effect, which, in principle, ought to be expected to be manifested in two different ways.

On the one hand, a thermoelastic effect - which is certainly conspicuous on concrete or brick bridges - is similar to what is observed on the Gran Sasso mountain data series (a massif in central Apennines) by AE records measured in a deep cavern (Paparo *et al.*, 2002; Gregori and

Paparo, 2004; Gregori *et al.*, 2012). This effect is the consequence of the cooling and/or warming of the shallower layers of the rocks (limestone and dolomia) of the mountain. This cooling or warming involves first the outer layer, and later on the deeper layers. When the body warms up, the outer layer experiences thermal expansion, while it overlies colder and thermally more contracted inner layers. In contrast, when the body cools off, the outer layer shrinks due to thermal compression, while the inner layers are still warm and more expanded. Hence, the outer layers have insufficient room, and some crack will occurs in the outer layer. The phenomenon is the same as what happens to the furniture of a non-heated house, during the cold early-morning hours in winter time. Or this is the same well known phenomenon which typically occurs to rocks in an extreme desert area, etc.

Since, compared to a metal, concrete and bricks have smaller thermal conductivity, the thermoelastic degrading is expected to be comparably more relevant in concrete or brick bridges. And this effect is likely to be maximum when the thermal gradient is comparatively larger during the *cooling* process, i.e. during the early hours of the day. This is the aforementioned effect observed on Gran Sasso.

In contrast, when dealing with a metal structure, a different behavior ought to be observed. The linear elongation of the large metal components of the bridge is the cause of large displacements of the supporting points of every bridge element (during the aforementioned Step 1 of the load test the bridge elongated by 11 mm). This phenomenon ought to be comparatively larger when the absolute value of either the warming or the cooling process is maximum. This maximum (cooling) occurs during the first few hours afternoon. This effect ought therefore to be comparatively more relevant on metal bridges, compared to concrete bridges. This is observed on the Garbatella bridge.

Therefore, whenever temperature records are eventually available during AE monitoring of a bridge, constructed either by concrete or by bricks or by wood or by metal, the temperature gradient ought to be considered, and the response of the AE signal is different depending on the thermal conductivity of the material.

Since violent time-variations of the LF AE signal occurred also during the days when the working activity was totally (or almost totally) absent due to Christmas holiday, the phenomenon ought to be only - or almost only - thermoelastic.

Consider that this thermoelasticity implications were here observed on a bridge in Rome, where a mild and temperate climate is normally enjoyed. The thermoelastic effect has therefore to be expected to be much more important, in terms of ageing hazard, in the case of a bridge located in some comparably more severe environment.

For completeness sake, the HF AE figure analogous to figure 11 is shown in figure 12, which plots raw HF AE data in a *24-hour* cycle diagram. In general, the AE signal was recorded only during the warmer hours of the day, when a thermoelastic effect was active.

Note, however, that after *Dec 16th*, ~ *21 p.m.* through *Dec 17th* ~ *6 a.m.* the viaduct was recovering after the heavy stress of roadbed deposition, and the AE signal was therefore conspicuous.

In addition, during *Dec 24*[th], between ~ *21 – 23 p.m.*, some environmental disturbances, i.e. likely wind gusts, caused detectable AE signals.

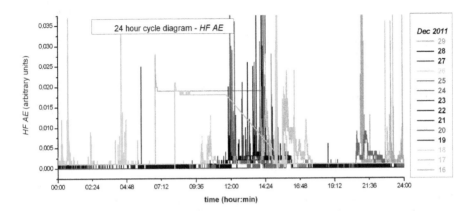

Figure 12. Raw HF AE data, *24-hour* cycle diagram. In general, the AE record were underflow except during the warmer hours of the day, when a thermoelastic effect was active. But, after *Dec 16*[th], ~ *21 p.m.* until *Dec 17*[th] ~ *6 a.m.* the viaduct was recovering after the heavy stress of roadbed deposition, and the AE signal was therefore conspicuous. In addition, during *Dec 24*[th], between ~ *21 – 23 p.m.*, some environmental disturbances, i.e. likely wind gusts, produced clearly detectable AE signals.

5.2. Wind gusts

Figure 13 shows a 24 hour cycle diagram of $D_t(t_j)$ of the HF AE *4 sec* data set. Figure 13 displays a comparably confused trend. There is, however, some large effect, which seems thermoelastic. Also the effect of hail is observed (see section 5.5). But, several most prominent disturbances appear uncorrelated either with Sun hours during the day, or also with working days, as during this period of time several days were total holiday. Hence, these disturbances are very likely to be associated with strong wind gusts that frequently, and more or less erratically, occurred during those days in Rome.

Therefore it is reasonable to conclude that wind gusts play a definitely relevant role in metal ageing, even on a bridge that has a structure which is likely to exert a limited aerodynamic opposition to wind.

The plot analogous to figure 13, but referring to LF AE is shown in figure 14, which is shown only for the sake of completeness. But no apparent regularity is observed. The trend appears definitely less influenced by the thermoelastic effect. The excellent performance of the viaduct is shown by the D_t values comprised between ~ 0.6 and ~0.95. But, during the afternoon some finishing works were being carried out, corresponding to lower D_t values. However, the anomalous low value of D_t occurred between *04:45* and *04:50* LT of *Dec 22*, and it clearly corresponds to a period when the LF AE was constant and underflow. Hence, as mentioned in section 5, it is found $D_t(t_j)=0$.

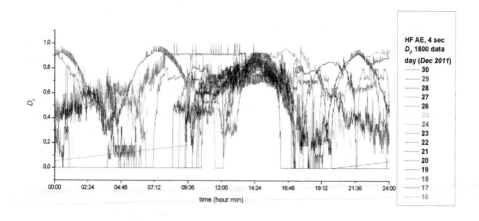

Figure 13. Superposed epoch representation (or "cycle diagram" for *24 hour* period) of D_t HF AE of the *4s* set. Colored lines are the date (*Dec 2011*). No offset was applied. The thermoelastic effect is clearly recognized during the early hours of every afternoon. The violent and erratic oscillations during all other hours of the day are the very likely consequence of strong wind gusts. The flat upper, almost linear, blue trend of *Dec 29* was caused by hail precipitation, and its superposed regular pattern of thin vertical lines is the oscillation of the viaduct at a period *~53.80 sec*. This same oscillation of the viaduct is also displayed like a sequence of thin lines at regular time intervals shown by several other lines in the present diagram. See text.

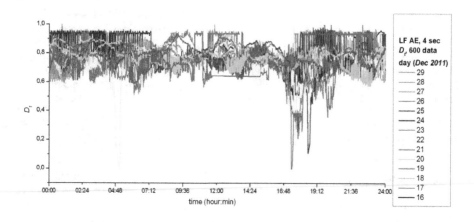

Figure 14. Figure analogous to figure 13, but referring to LF AE. The trend appears definitely less influenced by the thermoelastic effect. The excellent performance of the viaduct is shown by the D_t values comprised between ~ *0.6* and ~*0.95*. But, during the afternoon some finishing works were being carried out, corresponding to lower D_t values, or the LF AE signal was underflow. See text.

5.3. Trains

Trains frequently transit under the bridge, moving either slowly (say at $<10\ km/hour$) or faster (say at $\geq 50\ km/hour$).

The disturbance caused on the bridge depends on train speed v according to the following approximate order-of-magnitude estimate. Call m the total mass of displaced matter. If one considers the air blast caused by the train, m is the air mass which is contained inside an air volume equal to the volume of the train. Instead, if one considers the impulse caused by the mass of the train while it crosses on the railway under the viaduct, m is the mass of the train.

In general, it appears more likely to associate the AE disturbance to the shock-wave by air blast, better than to the soil shock caused by train's load. But, if an anemometer is available on the bridge, this dilemma can be promptly solved (see below). In any case, in either case the same following approximate argument can apply.

The impulse on the bridge is proportional to mv, where v is the train speed, and it occurs during a time lag which is roughly proportional to time spent by the train while it crosses under the bridge. If the length of the train is L , this time lag is $\Delta t = L\ /v$. Hence, the intensity of the effect which acts on the bridge may be defined as $F \propto \frac{mv}{\Delta t} = \frac{m}{L}\ v^2$. Therefore, a train that moves, say, at a speed $\geq 50\ km/hour$ causes an effect which is ≥ 25 times the effect of a train that moves at a speed of $10\ km/hour$.

The effect of the train can be clearly recognized in the $1s$ set, but only for HF AE (figure 15), and not in the LF AE (not here shown). This is consistent with the fact that this disturbance is feeble, in terms of consequences on the ageing of the crystalline structures. Hence, only some feeble transient signal is observed and clearly recognized only in HF AE. Differently stated, the disturbance originated by the transit of a train under the bridge is certainly less relevant compared either to wind gusts, or to diurnal thermoelastic effects, or to traffic load.

It is found that urban metro trains produce no sensible effect, as they move very slowly due to their regular stop at the Garbatella station. Only the suburban trains eventually transit at a comparably higher speed, and may cause a detectable effect. Consider also that the train crosses under the bridge at a level which is comparable with the entry of a high-speed train into a tunnel.

According to the official time table, which is reasonably correct (at most apart an error of very few minutes), suburban trains crossed under the bridge at the following times (for comparison purposes, their times have been transformed into day units and decimal fraction of a day). The times of the three trains that caused an HF AE effect are evidenced in bold: 20.50938, **20.51146**, 20.51979, 20.52188, 20.53021, **20.53229**, 20.54063, 20.54271, 20.55104, 20.55313, 20.56007, 20.56146, **20.56701**, 20.57188. The duration of the HF AE disturbance is consistent with the time lag spent by the train to cross underneath the bridge. For instance, a train (say) $\sim 50\ m$ long, moving at $\sim 50\ km/hour$, spends $\sim 1/1000\ hour$ to cross underneath the bridge. Hence,   the   perturbation   originated   by   the   train   ought   to   last $\sim 5 - 10\ sec \sim 0.002 - 0.003\ hours$. Tick marks in figure 15 are indicated every $0.005\ hours$.

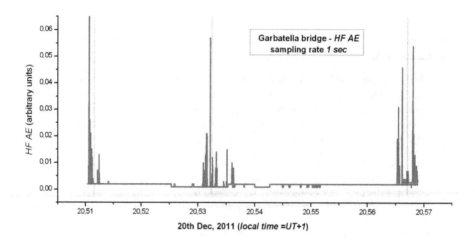

Figure 15. The effect of the train can be clearly recognized in the *1s* set, HF AE. The vertical green lines indicate the times, according to the official timetable, of the transit of every train that is likely to be responsible for an observed HF AE disturbance. Several other trains, with transit time in between these three "fast" trains, caused no HF AE disturbance, and were likely to have a much lower speed. See text.

If the air blast of a train is responsible for this effect, a similar effect ought to be observed for a wind gust. Hence, an anemometer located close to the bridge - and also close to its western terminal, where the railway is located and were the AE records were collected; see figure 1 - should clearly evidence the role of a perturbation on the bridge that is caused either by a wind gust or by a blast-wave by a train.

This datum is interesting for high-speed railways. When a high-speed train (with $v \sim 300 - 400$ *km/hour*) enters or leaves a tunnel, the impact of its shock-wave is $\sim 900 - 1600$ times the impact of the shock-wave caused by a train with $v \sim 10$ *km/hour*. This is responsible for a conspicuous ageing of the nacelle of the train. But, the same shock is applied also to the walls of the tunnel, which thus also experiences a corresponding ageing and potential security performance.

5.4. During the load-test

Figure 16 shows $D_i(t_j)$ during load-test. For comparison purposes both HF AE and LF AE are plotted in the present and in the following figures. The correlation appears evident with the sequence of "load-A", "load-B" and "load-C" sets. In particular, while the bridge was recovering after the stress originated by the "load-A" set, a new stress was applied by the "load-B" set, etc.

Figure 17 shows the same plot during a longer time interval, including $D_i(t_j)$ also during *Dec* 16th, when the bridge suffered by a violent stress caused by roadbed deposition.

5.5. Hail

Figure 17 also shows a much anomalous effect close to *Dec 17*[th], *10*[h] *43*[min] (=*17.44652* in day units). The cause was a short-duration hail storm (according to direct observation by the authors). The effect of hail grains is very small on the crystal bonds of the metal micro-structure of the bridge. While the hail storm is in progress, a tinkle is listened. But the AE transducer can record no audible signal. Rather it measures only HF AE and LF AE released by micro-crystal bonds, which are stressed and broken by hail's impact. However, owing to the very feeble intensity of the effect, the time sequence of the AE records responds essentially only to the timing of different hail grains that hit the bridge at different sites. Hence, since these gentle strokes are essentially random, it must be expected to find $D_t(t_j) \cong 1$, which is indeed observed. Note that other similar $D_t(t_j) \cong 1$ periods of time were observed in those weeks, when additional hail storms occasionally happened in Rome.

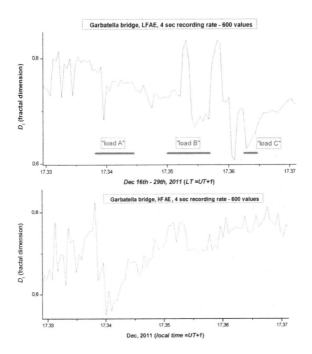

Figure 16. [upper plot] LF AE $D_t(t_j)$ during load-test. The correlation appears evident with the sequence of "load-A", "load-B" and "load-C" sets. [lower plot] HF AE $D_t(t_j)$ during load-test plotted for comparison purpose.

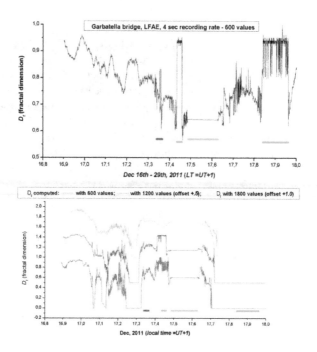

Figure 17. LF AE and HF AE $D_t(t_j)$ until *Dec 18th*. The horizontal bars at the bottom of the two plots indicate: the red bar the time of load test (from its beginning through its maximum load); the light blue bar the period of time with power supply failure; and the green bar the periods of time with hail precipitation. The lack of any $D_t(t_j)$ value for HF AE in the lower plot during the second hail storm (second green line) was caused by instrumental underflow. See text.

6. The proper oscillations of the bridge — The "*arp*" analysis of the outlier series

An interesting inference is derived by means of the "*arp*" of either HF AE's or LF AE's outlier time series, as shown in figures 18 through 21.

In the LF AE (figures 20 and 21) very clear evidence is found for two oscillations, the largest one with period ~ *20.324 min*, and a comparably smaller oscillation at ~ *53.798 sec.*[12] According to model computations, the first 4 proper oscillations of the viaduct, are, in decreasing order, *0.63 Hz*, *1.01 Hz*, *1.23 Hz*, and *1.29 Hz*.

---

12 In principle, every possible resonance of a viaducts ought to be avoided as far as possible. In this respect, the timing of the cross-lights, which control the access to the viaduct of the surrounding much heavy city-traffic, ought to avoid multiples or submultiples of this period, in order to prevent a possible effect by the impact altogether of a large number of cars on either one 3-lane way of the bridge.

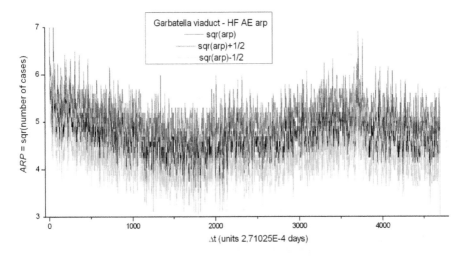

Figure 18. *"Arp"* for HF AE. It displays two major peaks at *1day 7.14348 min* and *1 day 27.43776 min*, respectively.

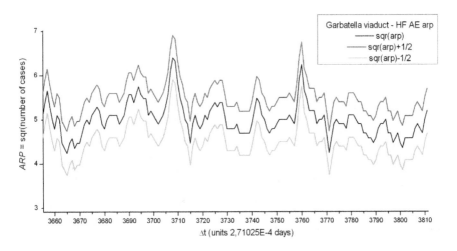

Figure 19. *"Arp"* for HF AE. Detail of figure 18, showing the two major peaks at *1day 7.14348 min* and *1 day 27.43776 min*, respectively.

That is, the two leading oscillation periods inferred by *"arp"* appear much different compared to model computation, although they are a clear and unquestionable observational evidence. On the other hand, consider that with one AE record every *4 sec*, or even every *1 sec*, it is impossible to search for frequencies close to ~*1 Hz*. Hence, a much higher time rate in AE

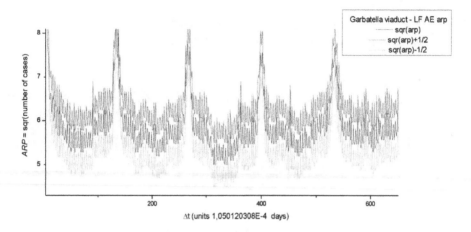

Figure 20. Lesser detail of the "*arp*" for LF AE, showing a major oscillation with period 20.323608 min. The full "*arp*" is not here shown, as it appears much regular and uniform, and it always displays the same periodical pattern.

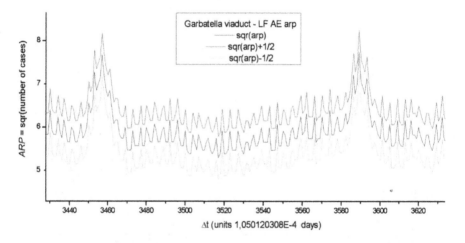

Figure 21. "*Arp*" for LF AE. Detail of the full "*arp*", clearly showing the second major periodicity at *53.7977869 sec*, which is also displayed by the entire "*arp*".

acquisition is strictly required in order to exploit a more pertinent check of the proper oscillation periods of a bridge with model computation.

It should also be pointed out that in the case of a volcano, e.g. of Peteroa (Ruzzante *et al.*, 2005, 2008), the analogous "*arp*" plot (unpublished) shows, unlike in the present case history, a dramatic superposition of very many different proper oscillation periods. Indeed, in contrast to every natural physical system, every manmade structure responds to a specific "simplicity" rationale, according to some ordered geometrical structure, etc.

The ~ 53.798 sec oscillation is also displayed in figure 13, although superposed over the large disturbances originated by wind gusts or by thermoelastic effects. It is also confirmed by the 1s data set. Figure 22 shows $D_t(t_j)$ for HF AE of the 1s set, computed by means of 600, 1200, and 1800 data. The N_D=600 case history oscillation appears closely correlated with the transit of the three "fast" crossing trains evidenced in figure 15. The most intriguing feature is evidenced by the N_D=1800 data case history, which displays a resonance oscillation with a frequency with period ~ 1 min (between 59.87 sec and 61.15 sec), to be compared with the aforementioned ~ 53.798 sec oscillation.

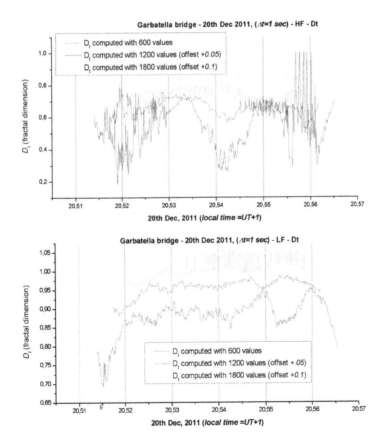

Figure 22. $D_t(t_j)$ for HF AE and LF AE of the 1s set, computed by means of N_D=600, or 1200, or 1800.

The same ~ 1 *min* period may be recognized also in the $D_t(t_j)$ LF AE *1s* data series, although only with *1800* data, and with a substantially larger scatter, due to the less faithful LF AE monitoring, compared to the HF AE monitoring, of the external applied disturbance.

In either case, consider that the *1s* set spans a short time interval, and the statistical dependence on N_D results dramatic.

As far as the HF AE are concerned, figures 18 and 19 display a large maximum of *"arp"* corresponding to the diurnal variation (two peaks at ~ 1 *day 7 min*, and ~ 1 *day 27 min*) which is evident in figure 6, although it is mainly a consequence of underflow of the AE detecting device. No other intuitively clear periodicities are evidenced, and are to be investigated by a specifically devoted investigation (in preparation).

7. Conclusion

AE monitoring of a metal viaduct appears much effective, feasible, and practical. The same procedure, apart lesser changes in procedures, can be successfully applied also to every concrete or brick or wood bridge.

The recommendations are here summarized, which ought to be taken into account when implementing an AE monitoring on a viaduct.

What parameter should be monitored?

LF AE are certainly much better suited to monitor the overall bridge performance. In general, HF AE may appear comparably less useful. However, HF AE can result important - or sometimes even crucial - whenever a more precise physical interpretation is needed while dealing with some unexpected or unwanted behaviour of materials.

In addition, regular records of meteorological and other environmental parameters ought to be monitored. Also the instant traffic load might be an important environmental information, although, in general, after a suitable calibration carried out once forever, the traffic signal is likely to be easily recognized by a simple routine AE monitoring alone.

What is the recommended time rate?

One rms time-averaged AE record, say, every *25-50 msec* appears to be a good choice, upon considering costs for instruments and data handling, and also the detail which is required in order to detect the proper oscillations of the viaduct.

By this, all kinds of hazard can be safely monitored (except an eventual very rapid damage, such as caused by an explosion, which should require a much higher time rate; but in general this information is of no practical interest).

What is the best procedure for AE monitoring?

In principle, AE monitoring can be operatively planned in three different ways: *(i)* steady permanent real-time monitoring operated from a remote control room; *(ii)* steady permanent monitoring with AE records stored by a data acquisition system, to be later recovered and analyzed; *(iii)* AE test carried out once-in-a-while either periodically or depending on particularly heavy environmental or traffic stress, etc.

The choice of either one procedure, or another, depends on costs and on the specific requirements by the user.

In general, real time remote monitoring may result less expensive, in terms of personnel and of routine automatic operation.

In addition, a once-in-a-while operation cannot be carried out on an instant basis. Indeed, in general one drawback is the time required by the AE recording apparatus to reach regime standard operation. In addition, environmental conditions, such as rain and subsoil water flow, may affect only on some days and not on others the long-term stability of a pillar of a bridge, etc. The same warning applies to every transient disturbance, such as wind gusts which occur only on some days, or a more or less intense diurnal thermal excursion, etc.

In addition, a real-time remote monitoring is also a warranty for a prompt alert about abrupt events that may severely affect the viaduct security (landslides, hurricanes, floods, terrorism, etc.).

How many AE devices are required on a viaduct structure?

In general one AE recording device is needed for every "monolithic" component of the bridge. By "monolithic" component it is here meant a unique solid body through which AE are effectively transmitted. For instance, a metal bridge is a unique huge metal body, and every AE, which is released at any point inside it, is promptly transmitted to all other parts of the bridge with negligible damping (at least as far as the size of the bridge in not exceedingly large).

In addition, the recommendations are to be taken into account provided by structural engineers, who should indicate the nodes that are likely to support the largest stress and are therefore the points that are more likely to suffer by a comparably more rapid ageing.

In any case, a given composite bridge in general has several pillars, and it is likely that AE cannot be easily transmitted from one pillar to the next. Hence, it is necessary to install an AE monitoring on every pillar. The same recommendation holds for every arch. In addition, suitable consideration ought to be given for the connection of a bridge to ground on either one of its sides, mainly whenever there is also a tunnel immediately close to the bridge, etc.

In general, AE monitoring ought to be recommended to be simultaneously operated at different points on the viaduct. However, it is also possible to envisage a periodical AE test carried out at different times and on different pillars, nodes, etc. Instrumental costs may be reduced, but operational costs may result to be largely increased, and the detail is certainly reduced of the final information about loss of performance and about security.

That is, every case history has to be considered independently, and the costs for implementation and operation are to be optimized depending on the required kind of alert which is required by the user.

What is the relevant difference between a metal viaduct and a concrete or brick or wood viaduct?

The aforementioned "monolithic" component structure has to be taken into account when dealing with every kind of viaduct.

Concrete bridges are expected to suffer by the comparative more intense thermoelastic effect during the early hour of a cold morning, unlike metal bridges that suffer by thermal excursion mainly during the hotter hours of the day.

A present great concern deals with the unknown performance of concrete, when it is older than one century, mainly when its ageing is combined with the effect of some particularly hostile environment.

Brick bridges ought to be tested in order to assess how far AE can be transmitted between contiguous bricks depending on the specific kind of mortar that was used. In general, a brick wall has a much compact structure, and in general AE transmission is likely to result much effective. In addition, in general a wetting of materials may dramatically improve AE transmission, etc. Hence, every case history has to be suitably evaluated, and every aforementioned warning has to be considered, which also applies to metal or concrete bridges.

Wood bridges require no particular additional warning, other than the investigation and calibration of that specific kind of wood, when it is strained by an applied stress. Compared to metal or concrete or stone etc., wood behaves much differently depending on its fibrous structure, which determines its "elastic" or "plastic" response, and also some kind of comparably time-delayed final yielding and rupture.

Acknowledgements

We thank Ing. Francesco Del Tosto for kindly providing us with some information about the height of the viaduct with respect to the railway, and about the preliminary activity on the bridge, carried out on *December 16th*, the day preceding the load test. We thank Ing. Fabio Rocchi for kindly providing us with the official documentation and drawings dealing with the load test of the viaduct.

Author details

Giovanni P. Gregori[1,2,3], Giuliano Ventrice[1,4,5], Sebastiano Pinori[1,6], Genesio Alessandrini[1,6] and
Francesco Bianchi[1,7]

*Address all correspondence to: giovanni.gregori@sme-ae-it

1 S.M.E. (Security, Materials, Environment) s.r.l., Roma, Italy

2 IEVPC – International Earthquake and Volcano Prediction Center, USA

3 IDASC(CNR), Roma, Italy

4 PME Engineering (Progettazione Macchine Elettroniche), Italy

5 SAE-Technology (System Acoustic Emission Technology), Italy

6 "Più s.r.l. costruire il futuro"- Gruppo Alessandrini, Italy

7 Faculty of Architecture, Third University of Rome, Italy

References

[1] Biancolini, M. E., Carlo Brutti, Gabriele Paparo, Alessandro Zanini, 2006. Fatigue
cracks nucleation on steel, acoustic emission and fractal analysis. *Int. J. Fatigue*, 28,
(12), 1820-1825.

[2] Braccini, S., C. Casciano, F. Cordero, F. Frasconi, G. P. Gregori, E. Majorana, G. Paparo, R. Passaquieti, P. Puppo, P. Rapagnani, Fulvio Ricci, and R. Valentini, 2002.
Monitoring the acoustic emission of the blades of the mirror suspension for a gravitational wave interferometer. *Phys. Lett. A*, 301, 389-397.

[3] Cello, Giuseppe, 2000. A quantitative structural approach to the study of active fault
zones in the Apennines (peninsular Italy), *J. Geodyn.*, 29, 265-292.

[4] Cello, Giuseppe, and B. D. Malamud, (eds), 2006. Fractal analysis for natural hazards,
Geol. Soc. Lond., Spec. Publ., 261, 1-172.

[5] Gregori, Giovanni P., and Gabriele Paparo 2006. The Stromboli crisis of 28÷30 December 2002. *Acta Geod. Geophys. Hung.*, 41, (2), 273-287.

[6] Gregori, Giovanni P., and Gabriele Paparo, 2004. Acoustic emission (*AE*). A diagnostic tool for environmental sciences and for non destructive tests (with a potential application to gravitational antennas), in *Schröder (2004)*, 166-204.

[7] Gregori, Giovanni P., Gabriele Paparo, Maurizio Poscolieri, and Alessandro Zanini, 2005. Acoustic emission and released seismic energy. *Natural Hazards Earth System Sci.*, 5, 777-782.

[8] Gregori, Giovanni P., Gabriele Paparo, Maurizio Poscolieri, Claudio Rafanelli, and Giuliano Ventrice, 2012. Acoustic emission (AE) for monitoring stress and ageing in materials, composing either manmade or natural structures, and their precursors. In *Sikorski (2012)*, 365-398.

[9] Gregori, Giovanni P., Gabriele Paparo, Ugo Coppa, and Iginio Marson, 2002. Acoustic emission in geophysics: a reminder about the methods of analysis. *Boll. Geofis. Teor. Appl.*, 43, (1/2), 157-172.

[10] Gregori, Giovanni P., Matteo Lupieri, Gabriele Paparo, Maurizio Poscolieri, Giuliano Ventrice, and Alessandro Zanini, 2007. Ultrasound monitoring of applied forcing, material ageing, and catastrophic yield of crustal structures. *Nat. Hazards Earth Syst. Sci.*, 7, 723-731.

[11] Gregori, Giovanni P., Maurizio Poscolieri, Gabriele Paparo, Sara De Simone, Claudio Rafanelli, and Giuliano Ventrice, 2010. "Storms of crustal stress" and AE earthquake precursors, *Nat. Hazards Earth Syst. Sci.*, 10, 319-337.

[12] Guarniere, Salvatore, 2003. L'emissione acustica come strumento diagnostico di strutture a varia scala. *Unpublished PhD Thesis*, 144 pp., University of Messina, Messina, Italy.

[13] Kapteyn, Jacobus Cornelius, 1903. *Skew frequency curves in biology and statistics*, Astronomical Laboratory, Noordhoff, Groningen.

[14] Kapteyn, Jacobus Cornelius, 1912. Definition of the correlation - coefficient. *Month. Not. Roy. Astr. Soc.*, 72, 518-525.

[15] Kapteyn, Jacobus Cornelius, and Marie Johan van Uven, 1916. *Skew frequency-curves in biology and statistics*, 69 pp., Hoitsema Brothers, Groningen.

[16] Lagios, Evangelos, Vassilis A. Sakkas, Issaak Parcharidis, Maurizio Poscolieri, Giovanni P. Gregori, Gabriele Paparo, and Iginio Marson, 2004. Ground deformation deduced by *DGPS, DInSAR, AE*, and *DEM* analysis in Cephallonia Island, presented at the *SCI 2004* congress, *The 8th World Multi-Conference on Systemics, Cybernetics and Informatic*, Orlando (Florida) 18-21 July, 6 pp.

[17] Paparo, Gabriele, and Giovanni P. Gregori, 2003. Multifrequency acoustic emissions (*AE*) for monitoring the time evolution of microprocesses within solids. *Reviews of Quantitative Nondestructive Evaluation*, 22, (*AIP Conference Proceedings* ed. by D. O. Thompson and D. E. Chimenti), 1423-1430.

[18] Paparo, Gabriele, Giovanni P. Gregori, Alberto Taloni, and Ugo Coppa, 2004. Acoustic emissions (*AE*) and the energy supply to Vesuvius – 'Inflation' and 'deflation' times. *Acta Geod. Geophys. Hung.*, 40, (4), 471-480.

[19] Paparo, Gabriele, Giovanni P. Gregori, Francesco Angelucci, Alberto Taloni, Ugo
      Coppa, and Salvo Inguaggiato, 2004a. Acoustic emissions in volcanoes: the case his-
      tories of Vesuvius and Stromboli. In the *Proceedings of the SCI 2004 meeting*, Orlando,
      Florida, July 2004.

[20] Paparo, Gabriele, Giovanni P. Gregori, Maurizio Poscolieri, Iginio Marson, Francesco
      Angelucci, and Giorgia Glorioso, 2006. Crustal stress crises and seismic activity in the
      Italian peninsula investigated by fractal analysis of acoustic emission (*AE*), soil exha-
      lation and seismic data. In *Cello and Malamud (2006)*, 47-61.

[21] Paparo, Gabriele, Giovanni P. Gregori, Ugo Coppa, Riccardo de Ritis, and Alberto
      Taloni, 2002. Acoustic emission (*AE*) as a diagnostic tool in geophysics. *Annals of Geo-
      physics*, 45, (2), 401-416.

[22] Poscolieri, Maurizio, Evangelos Lagios, Giovanni P. Gregori, Gabriele Paparo, Vassi-
      lis A. Sakkas, Issaak Parcharidis, Iginio Marson, Konstantinos Soukis, Emmanuel
      Vassilakis, Francesco Angelucci, Spyridoula Vassilopoulou, 2006. Crustal stress and
      seismic activity in the Ionian archipelago as inferred by combined satellite and
      ground based observations on the Kefallinìa Island (Greece). In *Cello and Malamud
      (2006)*, 63-78.

[23] Poscolieri, Maurizio, Giovanni P. Gregori, Gabriele Paparo, and Alessandro Zanini,
      2006a. Crustal deformation and *AE* monitoring: annual variation and stress-soliton
      propagation, *Nat. Hazards Earth Syst. Sci.*, 6, 961-971.

[24] Ruzzante, Josè, and Maria Isabel Lòpez Pumarega, (eds), 2008. *Acoustic emission*, Vol.
      1, *Microseismic, learning how to listen to the Earth…*, 68 pp., CNEA, Buenos Aires. ISBN
      978-987-05-4116-5.

[25] Ruzzante, José, Gabriele Paparo, Rosa Piotrkowski, Maria Armeite, Giovanni P. Gre-
      gori, and Isabel Lopez, 2005. Proyecto Peteroa, primiera estaciòn de emisiòn acustica
      en un volcàn de los Andes, *Revista de la Uniòn Iberoamericana de Sociedades de Fìsica*, 1,
      (1), 12-18.

[26] Ruzzante, Josè, Maria Isabel Lòpez Pumarega, Giovanni P. Gregori, Gabriele Paparo,
      Rosa Piotrkowski, Maurizio Poscolieri, and Alessandro Zanini, 2008. Acoustic emis-
      sion (*AE*), tides and degassing on the Peteroa volcano (Argentina). In *Ruzzante and
      Lòpez Pumarega (2008)*, 37-68.

[27] Schröder, Wilfried, (ed.), 2004. Meteorological and geophysical fluid dynamics (A
      book to commemorate the centenary of the birth of Hans Ertel), 417 pp., *Arbeitkreis
      Geschichte der Geophysik und Kosmische Physik*, Wilfried Schröder/Science, Bremen.

[28] Sikorski, Wojciech, (ed.), 2012. *Acoustic emission*, 398 pp., InTech; *http://www.intechop-
      en.com/articles/show/title/acoustic-emission-ae-for-monitoring-stress-and-ageing-in-materi-
      als-including-either-manmade-or-natur*; ISBN 978-953-51-0056-0.

Chapter 6

Power Transformer Diagnostics Based on Acoustic Emission Method

Wojciech Sikorski and Krzysztof Walczak

Additional information is available at the end of the chapter

1. Introduction

Partial discharge (PD) diagnostics is a proven method to assess the condition of a power transformer. Too high level of PD in a transformer may quickly degrade its insulation system and lead to damage. If PDs are detected and located quickly, then the transformer may be repaired or replaced, thus preventing power outages (Bartnikas, 2002; Gulski & Smitt, 2007).

Partial discharges in power transformers in service are most often detected with DGA (Dissolved Gas Analysis) and afterwards located using acoustic emission method (AE) (Duval, 2008; Lundgaard, 1992; Bengtsson & Jönsson, 1997).

In regard to the possibility of location of defects generating partial discharges, acoustic emission is an important diagnostic method of power transformers and other HV equipment.

Widely applied techniques for the fault location based on AE method are: (i) measurement of the time difference of arrival (TDOA) of the acoustic signals, (ii) measurement of the acoustic signal amplitude in different areas of a transformer tank (standard auscultatory technique, SAT), (iii) advanced auscultatory technique (AAT), (iv) estimation of the direction of arrival (DOA) of the acoustic signal based on the phased-array signal processing (Markalous et al., 2008; Tenbohlen et al., 2010; Qing et al., 2010).

More and more frequent breakdowns of large power transformers, often ending with fire difficult to put out, compel to more critical evaluation of traditional diagnostics techniques based mostly on periodic testing. Ageing of network infrastructure causes that the possibility of insulation system damage resulting from defect developing in short period is becoming more and more real. This fact favours different kinds of monitoring systems, which, through continuous investigation of the most important transformer parameters, allow to early detection of coming damage.

While analysing described in the literature cases of damage of power transformers, one can observe that many of them were related to accelerated degradation of insulation system, caused by high activity of different kinds of partial discharges (Höhlein et al., 2003; Lundgaard, 2000). Therefore the PD intensity monitoring as well as monitoring of its dynamics changes in time, in selected, neuralgic points of transformer seem to be a very important indicator informing on coming damage.

Currently there are only a few commercial systems for partial discharge monitoring in the power transformer in the world. These systems are based on the method of measuring AE (*Acoustic Emission*) or UHF (*Ultra High Frequency*) signal and offer limited capabilities (Markalous et al., 2003; Rutgers et al., 2003). A drawback of these systems is that as autonomous devices they do not cooperate with superior systems, and only transmit information or alerts about the status of the unit, what makes difficult a subsequent analysis of the causes of failure and looking for correlation with other parameters recorded by the monitoring system of the transformer.

Project assumptions of the partial discharge online monitoring system, developed at the Institute of Electric Power Engineering of Poznan University of Technology, were quite different. The system was, of course, so designed and constructed that it can work as a standalone device, what corresponds to the demand on emergency short-term monitoring (e.g. by day or a few days). However, the authors designing device have made all effort to ensure that it can be also integrated with any system of full monitoring of the transformer, such as e.g. Mikronika SYNDIS ES, which has already been installed on tens transformers in the European transmission networks. Through open collaboration of systems, the data collected by the PD monitoring system are visible in the superior system, so that it is possible to perform a full correlation analysis with other recorded parameters (load, voltage, oil temperature, OLTC operations etc.). The first prototype implementation of the integrated system for PD monitoring and SYNDIS ES was performed on one of the power substations. Currently the authors have already got the annual experience related to the work of the system, what will be discussed later in the chapter.

2. Superior power transformers monitoring system — *Mikronika SYNDIS ES*

In the power transformer monitoring Mikronika SYNDIS ES system, which has been installed on a few substations, the functionality of the expert system was acquired due to implementation of the knowledge base consisting of mathematical functions and models of phenomena occurring in a power transformer. Basing on logical operations and implemented inference rules, the expert functions generate (in online mode) summary alarms, emergency signals and prompts for substation staff. Expert functions assign specific logical value to the rules and relations contained in the knowledge base. On their basis, the transformer condition is defined as *Normal, Warning, Alarm* or *Emergency*. The simulating calculations conducted in real-time are significant elements of evaluation of power transformer condition. Therefore, the specialized mathematical model of thermal state was elaborated basing on the elementary relations presented in the *IEC 60076-7 – Part 7: Loading guide for oil-immersed power transformers*. The model includes relation between load losses and the temperature mean of the separate bushing and tap changer position. The model was expanded on the work of the three power transformer coils as well as the relation between cooling effectiveness and number of working coolers or radiator batteries was included in the model. Basing on simulations, possibilities of a power transformer load at the current surroundings temperature are calculated every minute. In order to efficiently manage the resources, besides load and temperature analysis one can distinguish the following thematic groups in the monitoring system:

- moisture content in oil,

- dissolved gas analysis,

- cooling system,

- on-load tap changer,

- bushings,

- partial discharges.

3. Partial discharge online monitoring system

The prototype system for partial discharge monitoring presented in this chapter is the effect of several years of research, the results of which have already been presented, among others in (Sikorski & Walczak, 2010; Sikorski, 2012). In the mentioned literature items one can find more information on project assumptions and criteria for the selection of individual components of the system.

The system works basing on the detection of acoustic emission pulses recorded by piezoelectric contact sensors (PAC WD), which are mounted on the transformer tank. A practical solution enabling easy mounting of AE sensor with a constant force to the tank is the use of special handles fitted with strong permanent magnets and such solution was used in the prototype. The preamplifier is also mounted in the handle. The amplifier and filters are located in standard 19-inch, fully screened industrial housing. From the conditioning module signals are transmitted to the acquisition module. Its integral element is a powerful workstation, based on multi-core architecture, with specialized software and ultrafast acquisition card installed. Procedures for the acquisition and analysis of data are implemented in National Instrument *LabView* programming environment and realized in real time. Acquisition module, like conditioning module, was placed in a separate screened industrial housing, compatible with mechanics standard 19-inch. The housing is waterproof and equipped with automatic temperature control system.

The system is designed for continuous, multi-month fieldwork, therefore specialized software allows not only for continuous registration of partial discharge activity, but also for correctness of the work of the system itself (e.g. temperature and humidity inside the enclosure or operation of electronic measuring circuits). The program is equipped with advanced data processing modules, which make it easier to evaluate events and noise filtering. In addition to the registration and calculation of basic PD parameters (like the number of pulses, their energy and amplitude), the program creates also event log, whose goal is to inform, with a specified frequency (service station or the superior system), about the work of the PD monitoring system or threat to the transformer resulting from the intensity discharge growth. External communication is provided using a GSM modem (with an additional antenna) or LAN/WLAN network. The second solution was used in case of cooperation with the superior system of transformer monitoring SYNDIS ES.

The schematic diagram of developed partial discharge on-line monitoring system, which was in detail described in (Sikorski & Walczak, 2010), was presented in figure 1.

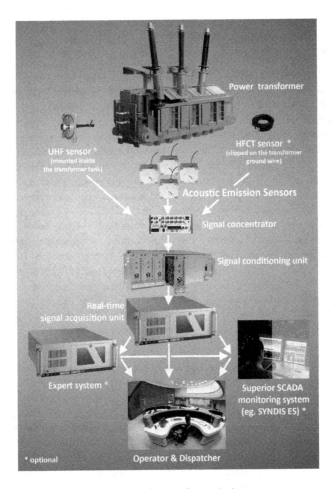

Figure 1. Schematic diagram of developed partial discharge on-line monitoring system

4. Partial discharge location techniques in power transformer

4.1. Standard and advanced auscultatory technique

Standard auscultatory technique (SAT) is one of the simplest methods of PD location. It involves the AE amplitude measurement in different areas of a transformer tank and thereby in different distance from the PD source. The SAT allows finding an area on a tank, in which the pulses of the highest amplitude/energy are recorded. One may assume that in this location under the surface of the tank, some depth in the object, the source of partial discharges' source is located.

The main advantages of the method are: (i) the possibility to carry out the measurements with one sensor, (ii) straightforward measurement procedure, (iii) the possibility of detection of the multi-source discharges, the occurrence of which in old transformers with aged insulation system is very probable (Sikorski et al., 2007, 2008, 2010).

Unfortunately, while employing the SAT method, very often one may expect errors in location of PD sources. This is because the amplitude of AE signal depends not only on the distance of a piezoelectric sensor from the discharge source (which is the basis of this measuring technique), but also depends on the energy fluctuations of partial discharges. Therefore satisfactory accuracy in the PD location with the SAT technique can be obtained only when discharges are stable (not self-extinguishing) and their energy does not change in time for the duration of the measurement. But taking into consideration that PD is a non-linear, dynamic phenomenon and has strongly stochastic character, this ideal situation is not very probable during the lengthy measurements performed on a real high voltage power transformer. The influence of small fluctuations of the PD energy on accuracy of discharges location with the use of standard auscultatory technique can easily be mitigated when one may determine the value of simple moving average (SMA) of the registered AE pulses' energy, e, and monitor the value of their standard deviation, σ. In case of fluctuations of the PD pulses' energy (e.g. their apparent charge q changes in a wide range, from hundreds pC to some nC), the procedure of AE-pulses energy averaging, does not give satisfactory results. The largest errors of the PD source location while employing the SAT method occur when the partial discharge activity is not-stable and after the period of high intensity we observe their extinction for a certain time.

In order to improve the efficiency and reliability of auscultatory technique, the authors propose to simultaneously monitor in each measuring point on the surface of a transformer tank the simple moving average of: (i) AE waveforms energy, $SMA(e)$, and (ii) the PD apparent charge, $SMA(q)$. Additionally, the parameter p is introduced that is equal to the quotient of the measured values $SMA(e)$ end $SMA(q)$. Due to this operation, the corrected value of the AE pulses energy depends mostly on the acoustic waves' attenuation effect, and so depends on the distance between a piezoelectric sensor and the PD source. The influence of the changes of PD energy on the result of the PD source location is then negligible.

The proposed algorithm of the AAT method consists of the following steps:

Step 1. Using the conventional electric method, identify the transformer phase, in which the partial discharges occur.

Step 2. On the transformer tank mark a grid of the measurement points, consisting of m-rows and n-columns (see Figure 2).

Step 3. For the given measurement point $a(i,j)$, where $i=1,...,m$ and $j=1,...,n$, simultaneously register r-values of partial discharge apparent charge $q=(q_1,q_2,...,q_r)$ and s AE-waveforms $X=[x_1,x_2,...,x_s]$.

Step 4. For the registered AE waveforms $[x_1,x_2,...,x_s]$ calculate their signal energy $e=(e_1,e_2,...e_s)$.

Step 5. For the registered values of the apparent charge $(q_1,q_2,...q_r)$ and the calculated AE waveforms energy $(e_1,e_2,...e_s)$ determine their simple moving average (SMA): $SMA(q)$ and $SMA(e)$.

Step 6. Calculate standard deviation σ of $SMA(e)$.

Step 7. If $\sigma \leq 0.1$ stop the acquisition, else repeat steps 3 through 6.

Step 8. Calculate the value of parameter p, which takes into account the influence of PD energy fluctuations on the energy of registered AE pulses in time for the duration of the measurements.

$$p = \frac{SMA(e)}{SMA(q)} \tag{1}$$

Step 9. Repeat steps 3 through 8 for all measurement points.

Step 10. Create matrix $P=[p_{i,j}]$.

Step 11. Create matrix $P_{norm}=[p_{normi,j}]$, which constitutes normalized values of matrix P in the range [0;1]:

$$p_{norm_{i,j}} = \frac{(p_{i,j} - p_{min})}{(p_{max} - p_{min})} \tag{2}$$

Step 12. On the base of the P_{norm} and the bilinear interpolation function generate a high resolution intensity graph (called *Acoustic Emission Map*).

Step 13. Superimpose the *Acoustic Emission Map* image on the photograph or construction drawing of the investigated transformer's phase, to find on the tank the areas which are the closest to the PD source.

Because the *Acoustic Emission Map* shows the result of PD source location on the 2D plane (see Fig. 3), it is recommended, if possible, to perform the additional measurements with the TDOA triangulation technique, by placing the AE sensors on the tank wall close to the area of highest p values localized with AAT.

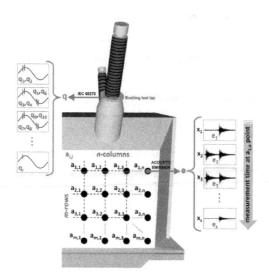

Figure 2. Schematic diagram of AAT measurement procedure

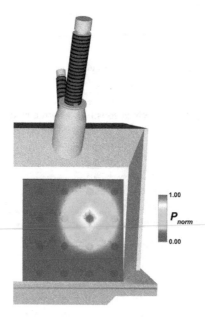

Figure 3. Two-dimensional visualization (*Acoustic Emission Map*) of PD-source location results in advanced auscultatory technique (AAT).

The most important modification, comparing to the SAT method, is application of the parameter p which, to a very significant degree, minimizes the negative influence of the temporal changes of PD energy on the defect location results. This positive feature is illustrated by a simulation shown in figure 4. For simplification, it was assumed that the defect is present in the 'B' phase of the transformer, and the AE pulses were registered only in 7 measuring points. In the first case, it was assumed that the partial discharges are stable and their energy does not change in time for the duration of the measurements. Of course, with such an idealistic and almost unrealistic assumption, both techniques achieve identical and correct result of the defect location (Fig. 4a). As for the second analysed case, when energy of PD varies (fluctuate) during the acoustic emission signals' measurements, only the AAT technique allows to obtain the proper location of the defect (Fig. 4b).

The on-site PD measurement using a standard IEC-60270 PD detector is complicated. There-fore, the new AAT method is dedicated mainly for the transformer manufacturing plants and the repair companies. However, modern PD-detectors with the integrated noise-gating channel for noise-suppression via an external antenna and the software for noise reduction and filtering may also expand the AAT usage to transformers installed at substation (Kraetge et al., 2010).

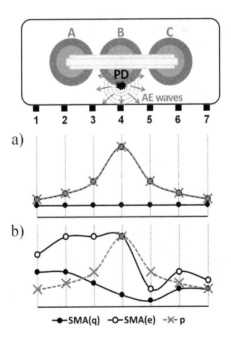

Figure 4. The diagram illustrating the result of PD location employing the parameter SMA(e) (standard auscultatory technique) and parameter p (advanced auscultatory technique) in case when the apparent charge of partial discharg-es is: a) stable, and b) varying in time during the measurement.

Due to a low sensitivity of the PD detection procedure using acoustic emission method, the AAT method is the best for location of the defects that are the source of discharges with high energy (e.g. surface and creeping discharges, sparks), or defects that are close to a transformer tank (e.g. discharges in bushing and near the winding at the bushing connection, on the surface of outer pressboard barriers and spacers, etc.). Unfortunately, location of the internal PD sources (e.g. within the winding), is very difficult or even impossible. It concerns not only the use of AAT method, but any other technique that is based on acoustic emission.

Furthermore, it should be stressed, that complex and non-homogeneous internal construction of the transformer (pressboard barriers, supporting beams made of wood or phenolic resin etc.) and transformer tank (corrugated walls, magnetic or non-magnetic shields, stiffeners, gussets or ribs reinforcing the mechanical strength, welds etc.) impedes a proper interpretation of the AAT results because it causes a strong suppression of the acoustic signal.

4.2. Time Difference of Arrival (TDOA) technique

The PD source location based on TDOA technique is usually applied during on-site diagnostic tests of large power transformers. At least four AE sensors are used for spatial location of a defect $PD(x, y, z)$ in transformer tank. The sensors theoretically are fixed in different distances from the PD source (Fig. 5). The position of the defect is estimated basing on measured time difference of arrival of acoustic signals. In order to find the coordinates of defect one should solve the following nonlinear system of equations:

$$(x - x_{s1})^2 + (y - y_{s1})^2 + (z - z_{s1})^2 = (v_{oil} \bullet T)^2 \tag{3}$$

$$(x - x_{s2})^2 + (y - y_{s2})^2 + (z - z_{s2})^2 = (v_{oil} \bullet (T + t_{12}))^2 \tag{4}$$

$$(x - x_{s3})^2 + (y - y_{s3})^2 + (z - z_{s3})^2 = (v_{oil} \bullet (T + t_{13}))^2 \tag{5}$$

$$(x - x_{s4})^2 + (y - y_{s4})^2 + (z - z_{s4})^2 = (v_{oil} \bullet (T + t_{14}))^2 \tag{6}$$

where: x, y, z – unknown PD-source coordinates in space, T – unknown acoustic wave propagation time from PD-source to the nearest sensor numbered as S1, $x_{S1...4}$, $y_{S1...4}$, $z_{S1...4}$ – Cartesian coordinates of the four AE sensors S1...S4, t_{12}, t_{13}, t_{14} - propagation time delay between the sensor 1 and the sensors 2, 3 and 4 respectively ($t_{12} < t_{13} < t_{14}$), v_{oil} – acoustic wave propagation velocity in transformer oil (1413 m/s at 20ºC, 1300 m/s at 50ºC, 1200 m/s at 80ºC).

This nonlinear system of equations can be solved with one of direct (non-iterative) solver algorithms or with a least square iterative algorithm, which efficiency strongly depends on initial values selected by user.

The most common errors in accurate location of PD source coordinates using TDOA technique in large power transformers result from:

- simplifying assumption that the acoustic wave propagates only in oil with the velocity v_{oil} < 1500 m/s. This ignores the fact that acoustic wave propagates in transformer tank wall with velocity 5100 m/s as well.

- incorrect time-of-arrival estimation of signal propagating along the shortest geometric path. In regard to the fact that the velocity in metal is greater than in oil, the acoustic wave, which most of its way travels in tank wall (structure-borne path), arrives at the sensor first. Afterwards the sensor registers the wave, which propagated in oil slowly (direct acoustic path).

- inaccurate measurement of coordinates of the AE sensors as a result of complex transformer tank structure.

Time-of-arrival of partial discharge pulses is usually estimated by an experienced expert. It is also possible to apply an algorithm dedicated for automatic time-of-arrival estimation (so-called auto-picker). Currently used algorithms giving satisfying results base on the following criteria: (i) Signal Energy (EC), (ii) Akaike Information Criterion (AIC), (iii) Discrete Wavelet Decomposition (DWT), (iv) Gabor centroid, (v) Maximum Likelihood (ML), (vi) Phase in frequency domain and (vii) trigger level.

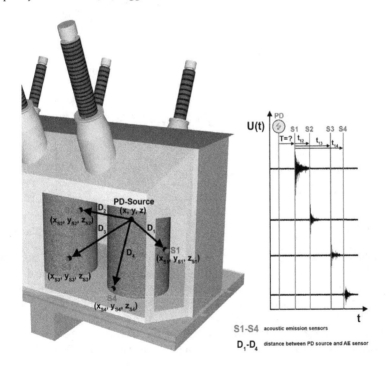

Figure 5. Schematic diagram of Time Difference of Arrival (TDOA) technique for partial discharge location in power transformer

In most cases, when signal-to-noise ratio (SNR) is high, the auto-pickers allow to estimate time-of-arrival with satisfying accuracy. In the rest of cases, it is necessary to apply additional advanced signal denoising methods, which increase the SNR.

The figure 6 presents the example of the time-of-arrival estimation of partial discharge pulse based on AIC and energy criterion.

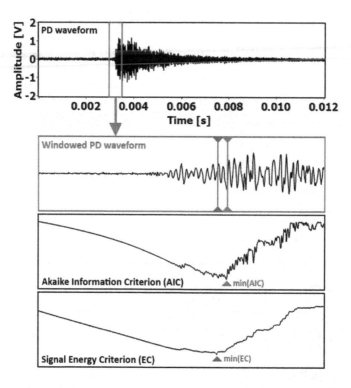

Figure 6. Exemplary estimation of the time-of-arrival of partial discharge pulse based on AIC and energy criterion

The application of triggering with an electrical (IEC-60270 detector, only in laboratory conditions) or an electromagnetic (RFCT or UHF sensors, both in laboratory and on-site conditions) partial discharge signal is another variant of defects location technique (Fig. 7). The main advantages of simultaneous use of electrical/electromagnetic triggering and acoustic emission method are: (i) obtaining information on time of partial discharge initiation and (ii) reduction in the number of AE sensors required for measurement procedure (three are sufficient). In order to locate PD-source the following system of equations should be solved:

$$(x - x_{s1})^2 + (y - y_{s1})^2 + (z - z_{s1})^2 = (v_{oil} \bullet t_1)^2 \tag{7}$$

$$(x - x_{s1})^2 + (y - y_{s1})^2 + (z - z_{s1})^2 = (v_{oil} \bullet t_2)^2 \qquad (8)$$

$$(x - x_{s1})^2 + (y - y_{s1})^2 + (z - z_{s1})^2 = (v_{oil} \bullet t_3)^2 \qquad (9)$$

where: x, y, z – unknown PD-source coordinates in space, $x_{S1...3}$, $y_{S1...3}$, $z_{S1...3}$ - Cartesian coordinates of the sensors S1...S3, t_1, t_2, t_3 – measured absolute arrival times, v_{oil} – acoustic wave propagation velocity in transformer oil.

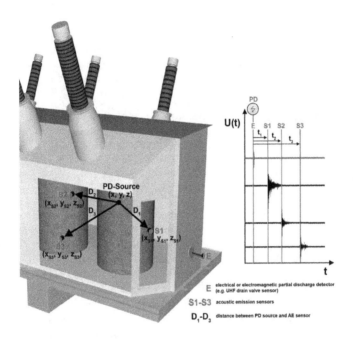

Figure 7. Schematic diagram of Time Difference of Arrival (TDOA) technique with electrical/electromagnetic triggering for partial discharge location in power transformer

5. Examples of partial discharge location and on-line monitoring

5.1. *Case study 1 —* Short-term monitoring (daily) of the 160 MVA transformer

Investigations were carried out in a power transformer 125000/220 manufactured in 1978 with the parameters shown in Table 1.

Parameter	Value
Type	RTdxP 125000/220
Voltage	230/120/10.5 kV
Power	160/160/50 MVA

Table 1. Main parameters of investigated transformer

The main reason for performing the partial discharge investigation was a disturbing level of flammable gases in the insulating oil, especially hydrogen. It was noticed just after a flashover which occurred in 2002 in a distribution line that caused a flow of the short-circuit current in the local power system. In successive years the periodic diagnostic measurements revealed a continuous increase of the amount of gases dissolved in the oil. In 2008 a sudden increase of gases in the oil was noticed. The amount of hydrogen exceeded the level of 2000 ppm, and the breakdown voltage of oil decreased to 18 kV, while the permissible value is not less than 50 kV for this type of transformer.

Unfortunately, even after oil treatment process, continuous increase of flammable gases in oil content was still observed. In 2009 SFRA (Sweep Frequency Response Analysis) investigation was made, and the results suggested that the axial displacement, as well as the radial buckling of low voltage and compensating winding was probable. In April 2011 the concentration of hydrogen exceeded 2200 ppm (with permissible value of 350 ppm), and content of CO_2 exceeded 3100 ppm, approaching the permissible value equal to 4000 ppm.

In order to estimate the danger of a transformer failure, the owner decided to make additional measurements of PD using the electrical method. For that reason, the 220/110 kV transmission overhead lines connected to this transformer had to be temporarily switched off. It should be noted that due to very intensive interference originating mainly from the corona on the transmission lines, it was not possible to detect the PD with the use of the conventional electrical method according to IEC 60270. However in this case, the substation was equipped with one transformer only, so when the transformer and the transmission lines were de-energized for the PD measurement system calibration, the interference did not exceed the level of 300 pC. Next, during the PD measurement procedure, when the transformer and the lines were switched on, the interference level changed from 400 pC (110 kV side) to maximum 8 nC (220 kV side), depending on investigated phase and transformer load. Measurements with the electrical method were done for all phases of the transformer (on 110 kV and 220 kV side) using the measuring taps of the bushings.

The measurement procedure was repeated for each transformer phase and consisted of:

1. Disconnection of transmission line and switching the transformer off,

2. Connection of the measuring impedance to the measuring tap of a bushing,

3. Calibration of the measuring system with the use of a standard PD calibrator,

4. Energization of the transformer and detection of the partial discharges.

Transformer phase	Apparent charge [nC]
HV 1	10
HV 2	17
HV 3	11
LV 1	N/A*
LV 2	1
LV 3	N/A*

* No PD activities or PD buried in background noise

Table 2. Maximum value of PD apparent charge registered during test

The result of the PD measurements carried out with conventional electrical method revealed the presence of strong discharges in phase *HV 2* (Table 2). The maximum value of apparent charge reached 17 nC (Fig. 8), however the range of a phase angle, in which the discharges appeared, was mainly from 30° to 90°. In other phases of 220 kV side (*HV 1* and *HV 3*) the PD pulses were also recorded, but their apparent charge value did not exceed 10-11 nC. The range of phase angle was identical as in *HV 2* phase. On the basis of the obtained results it was concluded that the signals observed in phases *HV 1* and *HV 3* were the same as those coming from the *HV 2*, but attenuated, indicating their origin as *HV 2*. In the case of 110 kV side, only the low-energy signals were registered with the apparent charge up to 1 nC, and in *LV 2* phase only.

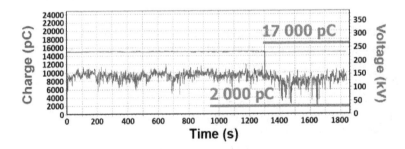

Figure 8. The results of PD apparent charge measurement in phase *HV 2* of investigated transformer.

On the basis of the results obtained with the use of conventional electrical method, it was decided that the procedure of PD source location should be restricted to *HV 2* phase only.

The time of investigation was not limited, as well as it was possible to carry out the continuous monitoring of the apparent charge level. It was also possible to perform the PD location using both the AAT and the TDOA triangulation.

In case of the AAT, in the first step, the measurement points on the surface of transformer tank were chosen and marked. These points formed a measurement grid. In order to increase the reliability of measurements, and simplify the interpretation of the obtained results, the fragments of tank walls with higher thickness were omitted (e.g. corrugated walls and welds). The measurement grid consisted of 36 points, as it is shown in figure 9a.

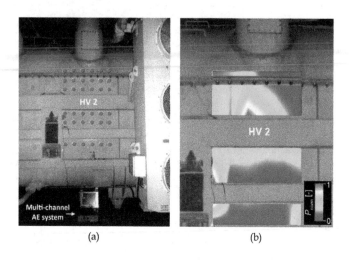

(a)   (b)

Figure 9. The measurement grid (36 points) used for PD source location with advanced auscultatory technique (a) and the result of PD source location presented as an *Acoustic Emission Map* applied in the picture of the *HV 2* phase of the investigated power transformer (b).

On the basis of the results obtained with the use of AAT, the *Acoustic Emission Map* was prepared and superimposed on a photograph of the transformer tank. The analysis of the *Acoustic Emission Map* image showed that in the HV phase 2 two sources of partial discharges were present (Fig. 9b).

When the acoustic emission measurements with the AAT were finished, a procedure of the PD sources location was initiated with the use of a triangulation technique. The AE sensors were placed on the tank wall in the locations identified by the *Acoustic Emission Map* image analysis. Placing the sensors in region of the strongest AE signals was done to increase the precision of XYZ coordinates' estimation of the PD source location using the triangulation method.

The analysis of the results of PD source location, obtained with the triangulation method showed that both sources of discharges were placed near the symmetry axis of the phase *HV 2* bushing and the transformer tank (Fig. 10a and 10b). On the basis of the investigation results, a hypothesis was assumed that partial discharges were generated inside the insulation of the winding leads or in the support beam that is close to the transformer tank.

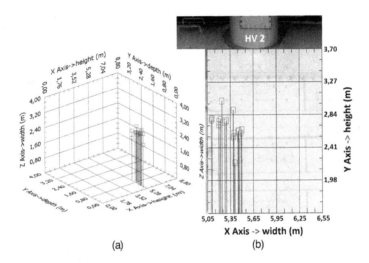

(a)   (b)

Figure 10. The result of the PD source location obtained with the use of triangulation method presented in the XYZ coordinates system (the XZ plane illustrates the wall of tank from the HV side) (a) and projection of calculated PD co-ordinates (XYZ) to the XZ plane (b).

Based on the obtained results of defect location and the analysis of the external structures of the transformer tank, the places, where acoustic emission sensors of monitoring system should be mounted, were selected (Fig. 9b). Due to the fact that AE sensors were placed close to located defect, on each of the four channels a similar number of acoustic events was recorded (Fig. 11). The amplitude of the signal recorded by each sensor was similar as well.

The same was also the average amplitude of the signal recorded by each sensor (Fig. 12). However, when looking at the distribution of number of AE events, it can be noted that daily activity profiles of the partial discharges recorded by pairs of sensor (00&01 and 02&03) were similar. This fact suggests the existence of two defects, which was already mentioned after the analysis of the location results with the use of *Advanced Auscultatory Technique* (see Fig. 9b).

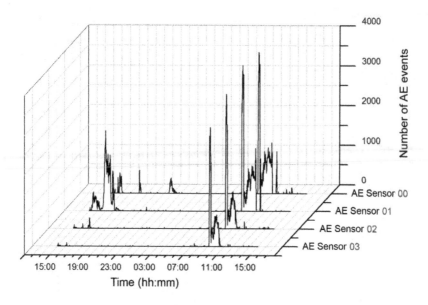

Figure 11. The number of AE events registered during daily monitoring of 160 MVA transformer

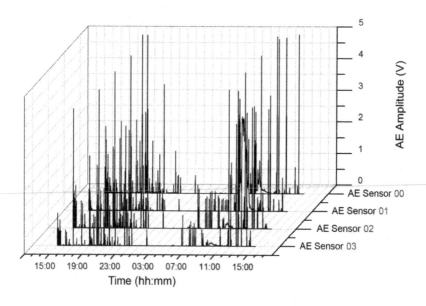

Figure 12. Amplitude of AE events registered during the daily monitoring of 160 MVA transformer.

Further interesting conclusions arise when comparing both the number of events and the average amplitude of the acoustic signal with daily load of the unit (Fig. 13). One can observe that the increase in the load is associated with increase of intensity and amplitude of partial discharges. Load peaks, occurring at 21:00 and 12:00, are accompanied by the largest PD intensity and highest average amplitude of registered acoustic signals. Probably, the temperature increased closed to defect, which was a consequence of the growth in the value of the current, causing intensification of the partial discharge phenomenon. Analysis of the impact of voltage changes caused by tap changes of the autotransformer, did not show any significant correlation with respect to the recorded acoustic signal (voltage change were small indeed).

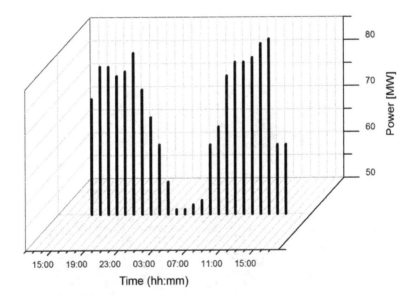

Figure 13. The value of daily load of the monitored transformer, registered in SYNDIS ES system

Observation of daily profile of PD activity changes also shows the advantages of on-line monitoring and imperfections of the standard approach to measuring partial discharges.

As one can observe in Fig. 11-12, the time of measurement can determine the quality of the analysis. During the day, both periods occurred in the monitored unit: extinction of partial discharges and their particular intensification.

Therefore one can conclude, that the choice of date and time for the implementation of periodic diagnostic tests by AE method (lasting usually no longer than a few hours) may have a fundamental importance for correct and reliable assessment of transformer insulation system. Of course, due to the stochastic nature of the partial discharge phenomenon, the most reliable results are obtained by monitoring the unit for a period of time at least one day.

5.2. *Case study 2* – Short-term monitoring (weekly) of 250 MVA transformer

A reason for installing the monitoring system to 250 MVA transformer was to observe from the beginning of 2011, the systematic increase of dissolved gases in oil (mostly hydrogen). The same year, in June, the location of the partial discharge sources by means of acoustic emission method was performed.

During the tests, several areas were located on tank in which recorded acoustic emission pulses were characterized by high amplitude. In the case of the lower voltage side (110 kV), repeatable pulses with the largest amplitude were recorded close to neutral point bushing (N). In addition, on the same side, sporadically occurring high amplitude PD pulses localized in phase *LV 1* and *LV 3* were recorded. During the measurements, any discharge pulses in phase *LV 2* were not registered (Fig. 14). In the case of the high voltage side (400 kV) sporadically occurring partial discharge pulses were also recorded, however, they were characterized by much smaller amplitude than it was in the case of the low voltage side.

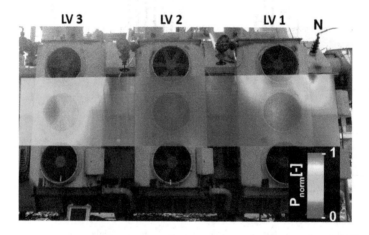

Figure 14. Results of PD source location (*Acoustic Emission Map*) obtained using advanced auscultatory technique (AAT) on low voltage side of the 250 MVA transformer

Due to further systematic increase in the level of hydrogen dissolved in oil and the alarming results of the detection and location of partial discharges, in December 2011 the transformer owner decided to install a monitoring system for a period of one week. Based on the results of the location, obtained before, three AE sensors have been mounted on the tank on the low voltage side near selected areas of greatest loudness (phase *LV 1* – sensor '02', phase *LV 3* – sensor '00', proximity to neutral point insulator – sensor '03'). The last sensor '01' was mounted in phase *LV 2* (as refer- ence sensor), where the test results showed that it is free from partial discharges. Such arrange- ment of AE sensors allowed the simultaneous monitoring of all phases of the transformer, with particular emphasis on critical points, which were fixed on the tank before. In the characteristics of the number of acoustic events registered during the weekly monitoring of the transformer were summarized in figure 15. In turn, on figure 16 the values of the oil temperature in top layer and voltages of monitored transformer registered in SYNDIS ES system were presented.

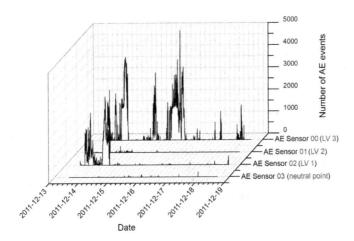

Figure 15. The number of EA events registered during the weekly monitoring of tested 250 MVA transformer

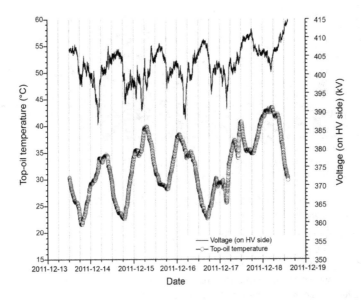

Figure 16. The value of the top layer of the oil temperature and voltages of the monitored 250 MVA transformer registered in SYNDIS ES system

Analysis of the characteristics showing the number of AE events recorded by the monitoring system confirmed the presence of partial discharges in phase *LV 1* and *LV 3* and the absence or presence of a few discharges in phase *LV 2* and close to neutral point bushing (Fig. 15). Monitoring showed that pulses with the highest intensity and energy are generated in phase C. The recorded PD pulses were unstable, and their ignition took place only in periods of voltage growth (Fig. 16). Moreover, it was noted that the moment of PD ignition correlates with temperature minima of top layer of oil, which may have a relationship with some dynamic changes in moisture at the interface of oil-paper insulation, described for example in (Borsi & Schroder, 1994; Buerschaper et al., 2003; Sokolov et al., 1999).

5.3. *Case study 3* — **Long-term (continuous) monitoring of 330 MVA transformer**

In this case the choice of the research object, on which continuous monitoring was tested, did not resulted from bad condition of the transformer. The primary purpose was integration of the PD monitoring system with the superior system (SYNDIS ES) and evaluation of opportunities for their cooperation. However, as in other cases, place of sensors location were selected basing on previously carried out detection and PD sources location using *Advanced Auscultatory Technique* (Fig. 17).

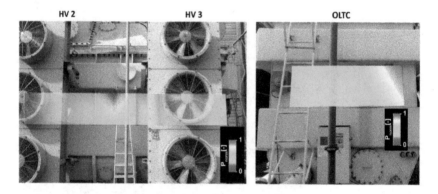

Figure 17. Results of PD source location (*Acoustic Emission Maps*) obtained using advanced auscultatory technique (AAT) on HV and OLTC side of the 330 MVA transformer

Acoustic sensors were installed in each HV-phase and on the tank of on-load tap changer (OLTC), in the place, where the pulses with the highest amplitude were recorded.

For the moment, the system worked continuously and without failure for about 9 months. At that time, it registered several periods of partial discharge activity, but their low intensity not suggested the possibility of a serious threat. However, the ability to correlate, e.g. the moment of PD initiation with different parameters recorded by the SYNDIS ES system (oil temperature, load, voltage etc.), seems to be interesting, especially from a scientific point of view and the possibilities for development and improvement of inference rules implemented in the software of monitoring system.

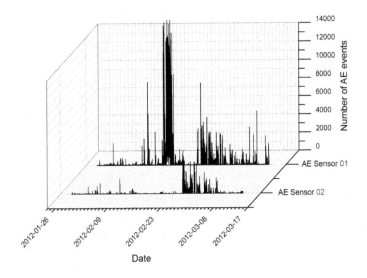

Figure 18. The number of AE events registered on 330 MVA transformer, where the long-term test of partial discharge monitoring system was carried out.

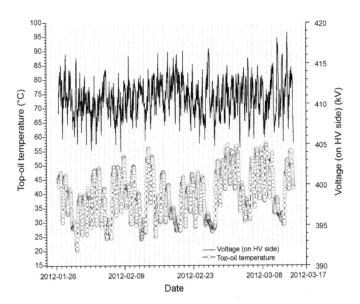

Figure 19. The oil temperature at top layer and values of voltages of the monitored 330 MVA transformer registered in SYNDIS ES system

For example, figure 18 shows the number of PD pulses registered by two sensors with numbers '01' and '02', installed respectively in phase *HV 1* and *HV 2*. As one can observe, partial discharges were transient, but comparison with other parameters, such as temperature and voltage (Fig. 19), allows to detect a correlation. As it was described in the previous case, the moment of PD initiation and growth of its intensity were connected not only with an increase in voltage, but at the same time, with relatively low value of oil temperature (20-30°C). Particularly high partial discharge activity has been reported in cases, in which the period of oil cooling and at the same time the growth of voltage lasted at least several hours. In the phase *HV 1* (sensor '01') this situation took place from 25 until 27 February, and in phase *HV 2* (sensor '02') between 12 and 13 day of the same month.

6. Conclusions

The chapter presents detailed description and features of the *Time Difference of Arrival* (TDOA) technique and new *Advanced Auscultatory Technique* (AAT) for location of partial discharge sources, as well as some examples of its practical application in power transformer diagnostics.

The developed by the authors *Advanced Auscultatory Technique* constitutes a synergistic combination of two diagnostic methods: (i) the acoustic emission (AE) and (ii) the conventional electrical PD detection method according to IEC 60270.

The presented research results proved numerous advantages of the AAT, among which the most important are:

- reduction of influence of partial discharge energy fluctuations on energy of registered AE pulses, which are the main reason of the PD source location errors with the standard auscultatory technique,

- clear and readable presentation of the fault location results in form of a high-resolution intensity graph (Acoustic Emission Map),

- the possibility of correlation between AE parameters and apparent charge,

- uncomplicated and quick PD location technique, particularly useful for transformer manufacturing plants and repair companies equipped with electrically shielded HV laboratory.

The partial discharge online monitoring in power transformer based on AE method was another important topic covered in the chapter.

The presented results largely confirmed the advantages offered by the partial discharge monitoring using the acoustic emission method, of which the most important are:

- ability to assess the profile of daily, weekly or monthly partial discharge activity,

- possibility of linking the partial discharge activity with other events or parameters recorded by the service station or other systems monitoring transformer work,

- ability to assess the dynamics of defect development,
- elimination of the interpretative errors which might arise in the standard and short-lived measurement procedures, and
- possibility of partial discharge sources location.

Author details

Wojciech Sikorski and Krzysztof Walczak

Poznan University of Technology, Poland

References

[1] Barnikas, R. (2002). Partial discharges. Their mechanism, detection and measurement, *IEEE Transactions on Dielectrics and Electrical Insulation*, , 9(5)

[2] Bengtsson, T, & Jönsson, B. (1997). Transformer PD diagnosis using acoustic emission technique, *10th International Symposium on High Voltage Engineering*, Montreal, Canada, August 1997, 25-29.

[3] Borsi, H, & Schroder, U. (1994). Initiation and Formation of Partial Discharges in Mineral-based Insulating Oil, *IEEE Transactions on Dielectrics and Electrical Insulation*, June 1994, , 1(3), 419-425.

[4] Buerschaper, B, Kleboth-lugova, O, & Leibfried, T. (2003). The electrical strength of transformer oil in a transformerboard-oil system during moisture non-equilibrium, *Annual Report Conference on Electrical Insulation and Dielectric Phenomena*, , 269-272.

[5] Duval, M. (2008). Calculation of DGA Limits Values and Sampling Intervals in Transformers in Service, *IEEE Electrical Insulation Magazine*, , 24(5), 7-13.

[6] Gulski, E, & Smitt, J. J. (2007). Condition Assessment of Transmission Network Infrastructures (April 2007), *10th International Symposium on High Voltage Engineering*, Montreal, Canada, August 2007, 25-29.

[7] Höhlein, I, Kachler, A. J, Tenbohlen, S, Stach, M, & Leibfried, T. (2003). Transformer Life Management, German Experience with Condition Assessment, Cigre SC12/AMerida-Kolloquium, June 2-4, 2003, 2.

[8] Kraetge, A, Rethmeier, K, & Kruger, M. & P. Winter, Synchronous multi-channel PD measurements and the benefits for PD analyses, *Transmission and Distribution Conferences and Exposition, IEEE PES*, (2010). , 1-6.

[9] Lundgaard, L. E. (1992). Partial discharge XIV. Acoustic partial discharge detection-practical application, *IEEE Electrical Insulation Magazine*, , 8(5)

[10] Lundgaard, L. E. (2000). Partial discharges in transformer insulation, *CIGRE Task Force 15.01.04*, Paper Paris, France, 2000, 15-302.

[11] Markalous, S, Grossmann, E, & Feser, K. (2003). Online Acoustic PD-Measurements of Oil/Paper-Insulated Transformers- Methods and Results, *13th International Symposium on High Voltage Engineering*, 978-9-07701-779-1Delft, Netherlands, August 2003, 324.

[12] Markalous, S, Tenbohlen, S, & Feser, K. (2008). Detection and location of partial discharges in power transformers using acoustic and electromagnetic signals, *IEEE Transactions on Dielectrics and Electrical Insulation*, 1070-9878, 15(6), 1576-1583.

[13] Rutgers, W. R. van den Aardweg P.; Aschenbrenner D. & Kranz H.G. ((2003). New On-line Measurements and Diagnosis Concepts on Power Transformers, *XIIIth International Symposium on High Voltage Engineering*, 2003, Netherlands

[14] Sikorski, W, Moranda, H, Brodka, B, & Neumann, R. (2010). Detection and Location of Partial Discharge Sources in Power Transformer, Electrical Review, 11b/2010, , 142-145.

[15] Sikorski, W, Siodla, K, & Staniek, P. (2007). On-line monitoring system of partial discharges occurring in power transformer insulation using acoustic emission method, *The 15th International Symposium on High Voltage Engineering*, Ljubljana, Slovenia, 2007

[16] Sikorski, W, Walczak, K, Siodla, K, Andrzejewski, M, & Gil, W. (2010). Online Condition Monitoring and Expert System for Power Transformers, *ARWtr2010International Advanced Research Workshop On Transformers*, Santiago de Compostela, Spain, 2010

[17] Sikorski, W, Ziomek, W, Kuffel, E, Staniek, P, & Siodla, K. (2008). Location and Recognition of Partial Discharge Sources in a Power Transformer Using Advanced Acoustic Emission Method, *Electrical Review*, 10/2008, , 20-23.

[18] Sikorski, W. (2012). *Acoustic Emission*, Intech Publishing, 978-9-53510-056-0

[19] Sikorski, W, Ziomek, W, Siodla, K, & Moranda, H. (2013). Location of Partial Discharge Sources in Power Transformers Based on Advanced Auscultatory Technique, *IEEE Transactions on Dielectrics and Electrical Insulation*, 2013

[20] Sokolov, V, Berler, Z, & Rashkes, V. (1999). Effective methods of assessment of insulation system condition in power transformers: a view based on practical experience, *IEEE Proceedings Electrical Insulation Conference and Electrical Manufacturing & Coil Winding Conference*, 1999, , 659-667.

[21] Tenbohlen, S, Pfeffer, A, & Coenen, S. (2010). On-site experiences with multi-terminal IEC PD measurements and acoustic PD localization, *IEEE International Symposium on Electrical Insulation (ISEI)*, , 1-5.

[22] Qing, X, Ningyuan, L, Huaping, H, Fangcheng, L, & Liheng, Z. (2010). A New Method for Ultrasonic Array Location of PD in Power Transformer Based on FastDOA, *International Conference on Mechanic Automation and Control Engineering (MACE)*, , 3971-3974.

[23] Qing, X, Xiang, X, Wang, N, & Fangcheng, L. (2010). Transformer partial discharge sources number estimation based on ultrasonic array sensors and modified CCT, *IEEE 9th International Conference on the Properties and Applications of Dielectric Materials (ICPADM)*, , 550-552.

Chapter 7

Testing of Partial Discharges and Location of Their Sources in Generator Coil Bars by Means of Acoustic Emission and Electric Methods

Franciszek Witos and Zbigniew Gacek

Additional information is available at the end of the chapter

1. Introduction

Although a leading role among testing investigations of partial discharges (PD) is attributed to electric methods [1], other complementary ones are developed permanently. One of them is acoustic emission (AE) method whose - using physical phenomena of AE - gives unique possibility to observe deformation processes [2,3]. Acoustic emissions have sufficient features so as to be an important measuring method, which may supply electric measuring methods of partial discharges. Basic disadvantages and limitations of acoustic methods (caused by changes of AE elastic waves generated by PD source during propagation within a medium, detection and handling data) can be eliminated by the choice of proper descriptors [4-6].

Authors are engaged in development problems of AE and its application for many years. During past years there were investigations of PD made by means of AE method. Authors worked out and built the original measuring system applied to record and analyze of recorded signals. The system is dedicated to testing of partial discharges by means of AE method. Measuring system enables us to record signals in real time within the band up to 500 kHz in laboratory and real conditions. Research method of acoustic signals bases on the software (written for this purpose); it enables us to describe signals and create AE descriptors. At present, the software contains programs for monitoring of signals, registration of data, basic and advanced analysis of registered data. This software can be developed if need be and creation of ideas concerning interpretation of measuring results will be created. Capability of the method designed to testing of AE signals, presented in the actual version, includes: filtration of signals within the given band, analysis of signals in domains of time, frequency and time-frequency, location of maximums at curves which are frequency characteristics of signals and averaging phase characteristics of signal modulus as well as testing of properties of amplitude distributions of an acoustic signal or a group of signals by means of AE method of descriptors, and finally - testing of properties of amplitude distributions of signal groups using Kohonen neuron network.

Authors made parallel testing of partial discharges in coil bars of the generator by means of AE and electric method. It is worth emphasis that results received from an electric method characterize the whole object - therefore they are global character. In turn, results received from AE method describe directly signals recorded at the given measuring point of the object (they are local character); connection of AE signals with these ones generated by AE sources needs knowledge of propagation conditions of AE impulses. Testing - carried out simultaneously - enable us to made independent analyses of described tested PD phenomena within a framework of particularly methods as well as to create description of phenomena common to both methods. Such a common description has an additional advantage - possibility to verify conformability of description received from both research methods.

2. The original system for recording of AE signals

In order to measure AE signals generated by PD, the original measuring system DEMA-COMP was designed and built [7,8]. It enables us to register signals in real time within the band of 20 - 500 kHz both in laboratory and real conditions. The measuring system contains four independently supplied measuring circuits. The maximum speed of 12-bit recording data to disk shall be 5 megasamples/second in each of the four channels. Software of measuring card was written in LabVIEW environment [9]. It contains programs for monitoring signals and registration data.

3. Basic analysis of recorded signals

Properties of recorded data in domains of time, frequency ad time-frequency are investigated in the frame of preliminary analysis of recorded signals. Analysis is made in the frame of activity of the program written for that purpose, named *AE+JTFA*. This program uses programming of LabVIEW environment.

Studied phenomena are of periodic and individual character. In view of the periodic nature of the investigated phenomena the authors analyze the recorded signals whose duration is many periods of the supply voltage – usually 2 seconds (i.e. 100 periods of the supply voltage). Particular signal characteristics are obtained over the periods of the supply voltage, and then averaged characteristics are calculated (Fig. 1).

In view of the individual nature of the studied phenomena (single deformation process), the authors perform an analysis of selected parts of the recorded signals.

Description resulting from analysis of an example AE signal whose time duration is 2 seconds (100 periods of supply voltage) is presented in Fig. 1. These results are as follows:

–signal after filtration with its minimal, maximal and RMS values (Fig. 1a); for filtration the band pass filter of 5 order is used, filtration band is given as a frequency range at the frequency characteristic,

–spectral power density as frequency characteristic of the signal with the frequency for main maximum and spectrum value for this frequency (Fig. 1b),

–phase-time characteristic (Fig. 1c),

–averaging phase characteristic (Fig. 1d),

–three-dimensional STFT spectrogram (Fig. 1e),

–three-dimensional STFT spectrogram dropped to a phase-frequency plane (Fig. 1f).

In order to obtain characteristics presented in Fig. 1, it should be determined filtration band first of all. Minimal, maximal and RMS values of the signal in volts are calculated by turns (Fig. 1a).

After filtration, the signal is put a next analysis in domain frequency, time and time-frequency. Analysis of the signal in domain frequency includes calculation of fast Fourier transform and power density spectrum as a square of complex Fourier transform. Additionally, the frequency for main maximum and value of the spectrum for this frequency in the spectrum is determined (Fig. 1b).

Within a framework of analysis of the signal in domain of time Authors worked out: phase-time characteristic of signal modulus (Fig. 1c) and averaging phase characteristic of signal modulus (Fig. 1d). The way how calculate characteristics in domain of the time is presented in Fig. 2. Phase-time characteristic of signal modulus (Fig. 1c and Fig. 2c) is obtained as follows: the signal selected for analysis is divided towards periods of the reference voltage (Fig. 2e shows the reference voltage during one of periods, Fig. 2f shows a signal recorded during the time determined in Fig. 2e), signal modulus (Fig. 2h) is calculated for each of periods and this modulus is placed on a phase-time characteristic as „two-dimensional section" (Fig. 2g). The phase-time characteristic of signal modulus (Fig. 2c) is created by „sewing" such „two-dimensional sections". This characteristic reveals periodic and random character of registered data. Averaging phase characteristic of signal modulus (Fig. 2d) is result of averaging of all„two-dimensional sections" (Fig. 2g) towards a phase of the reference voltage.

Analysis in time-frequency domain is based on JFTA analysis (*Joint Time-Frequency Analysis*) of the firm National Instruments [9]. The base is calculation STFT spectrogram (*Short-Time Fourier Transform*) or Gabor spectrogram for successive fragments of a signal of reference voltage. Authors worked out a new three-dimensional form of spectrograms, where time has been replaced by a phase of reference voltage. These spectrogram are calculated as follows. First of all it should be calculated three-dimensional spectrograms for signals registered in successive period of reference voltage. Finally, one should calculate averaging spectrogram of the signal (Fig. 1e), resultant from all spectrograms calculated for successive periods of reference voltage, as well as its projection on phase-frequency plane (Fig. 1f). Such a presentation facilitates location of PD on phase-frequency plane

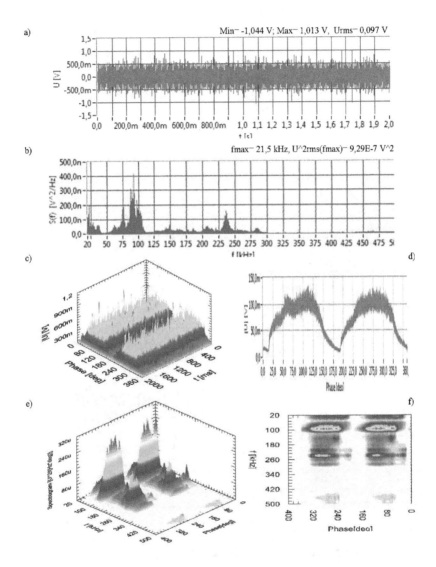

Figure 1. Introductory description of the example AE signal: a) impulse (after filtration), b) frequency characteristic, c) phase-time characteristic, d) averaging phase characteristic, e) and f) averaging STFT spectrograms; AE signal recorded in the following measuring conditions: measurement by means of WD sensor placed at P2 measuring point of „D" bar, the supply voltage of the bar 25 kV, measured value of the apparent charge 2.2 nC

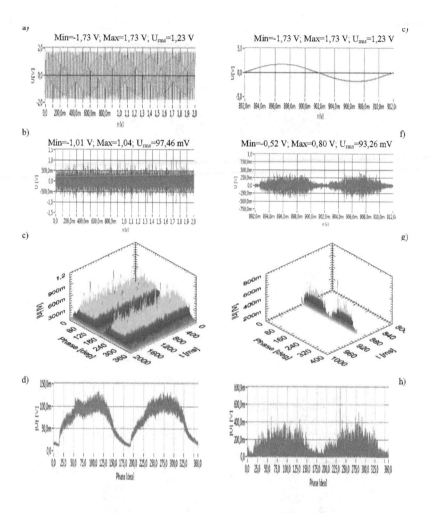

Figure 2. Preliminary analysis of registered data in time domain (for the signal from Fig. 1): a) reference voltage, b) signal after filtration, c) phase-time characteristic of signal modulus, d) averaging phase characteristic of signal modulus, e) reference voltage, f) fragment of signal registered during time given at the Fig. 2e, g) phase-time characteristic of signal modulus from the Fig. 2f, h) phase characteristic of signal modulus from the Fig. 2f

4. Advanced analysis of recorded signals

Within a framework of advanced analysis concerned recorded signals it is necessary to investigate recorded data in domain of discrimination threshold. This analysis includes calculation of amplitude distributions of AE signal power and AE counts in order to investigate their properties by means of the method of AE descriptors. Amplitude distributions of recorded signals are calculated by means of „AE+JTFA" program and next are visualized by means of other program named „AE amplitude distributions and descriptors", written for such a purpose.

Properties of amplitude distributions of AE counts and the power of AE signal (made in logarithmic scale) can be described by means of specially defined AE descriptors. The descriptors were defined as follows. At first, one should to mark a fragment of amplitude distribution curve which corresponds with the range of discrimination threshold (U_d, U_g); value of U_d is determined by minimum of derivative of distribution against discrimination threshold, whereas U_g is 90% of maximal value of recorded signal. Determined fragment of the curve is approximated by a straight line:

$$\ln(dN(U)/dt) = AU + B; \quad A = ADC \tag{1}$$

whereas the descriptor connected with the distribution is equals to slope of the straight A.

Described idea how define a descriptor for amplitude distribution of the power of AE signal is presented in Fig. 3. Descriptors defined in such a way are the base of the original advanced analysis of signals ascribing to acoustic emission signals AE descriptors with acronyms ADP (*Amplitude Distribution of Power of AE signal*) and ADC (*Amplitude Distribution of AE Counts*). Descriptors are calculated by means of the program „AE amplitude distributions and descriptors".

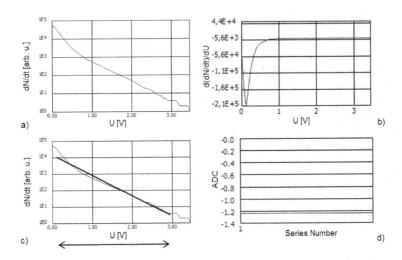

Figure 3. Illustration of ADC descriptor method calculation: a) amplitude distribution of counting rate, b) derivative of amplitude distribution of counting rate, c) amplitude distribution of counting rate with approximation curve and range of discrimination threshold (U_d and U_g), d) ADC descriptor for amplitude distribution from Figure 3a

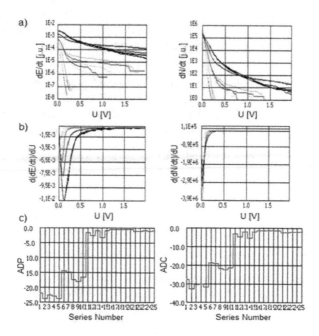

Figure 4. Test results concerned amplitude distributions made by means of the method of descriptors obtained with the program *Amplitude distributions and AE descriptors*: results for signal families recorded in measuring conditions differential only by applied voltages: U=10 kV (series 1-5), U=15 kV (series 6-10), U=20 kV (series 11-15), U=25 kV (series 16-20), U=30 kV (series 21-25))

Application of logarithmic scale on amplitude diagrams enables us to distinguish phenomena connected with propagation of an elastic wave in a medium and within an interconnected layer. Proposed definition of a descriptor and ascription of its value as the slope of a straight line, which approximates a chosen fragment of amplitude distribution, causes that descriptors are not based on values measured directly. Descriptors are negative values, and it is important that greater value of a descriptor is conform with flatter fragment of an amplitude distribution. Authors describe this property of defined descriptors as the so called advanced degree of AE signal, assuming that higher advanced degree of a signal is tantamount to greater value of a descriptor. Furthermore, Authors joint defined advanced degree of a signal with known advanced degree of deformation processes according to a rule that advanced degree of deformation process is described by AE signal generated in a source, whereas advanced degree of AE signal is described by a signal recorded at a measuring point (which is changed along propagation path). Test results concerned properties of amplitude distributions by means of the method of descriptors, for an example family of AE signal, is presented in Fig. 4. Authors have verified correctness of given hypothesis by analysis how are properties of many families of AE signals using the proposed method of descriptors [4,5,7,8].

5. Tested objects and description of tests

Tested objects were coil bars of the generator 120 MW, U_N = 13.8 kV (with outside control of electric field distribution [10]) and coil bars of the generator 200 MW, U_N = 15.76 kV (with outside and inside control of electric field distribution [10]).

Several hundred of generator coil bars are produced yearly in Poland. Each of these bars, before issuing of permit to work, is applied qualification tests. One of these tests consists in determination of PD level, carried out by means of electric method. Order of magnitude of admissible apparent charge in the case of considered objects is an order of nanoCoulombs.

Generator coil bar is a very interesting test object [11-15] because:

a.   it is a complex insulating system (electrodes, semiconductor areas to control electric field distribution, complex insulating and conducting layers) where different PD sources typical for solid materials may appear,

b.   AE sensors can be installed at many points of a tested bar which creates possibilities for identification of AE signals and location of PD sources.

Generator coil bars, produced by one of the factory, have been tested by means of AE method (using the original measuring system DEMA-COMP) and by means of electric method (using the computer measuring system TE 571 [8,16]). The purpose of these tests was analysis of PD phenomena appeared within generator coil bars resultant from two above methods applied simultaneously.

Within a framework of preparation for testing with the help of AE method it has been establish that tests concern only a slot part of the bar. This area is limited by additional earthed electrodes; between them there are six evenly distributed measuring points P1, P2,..., P6 (Fig. 5).

AE sensors (R6 and WD type, coming from the firm PAC[17]) have been placed at measuring points. Each tested bar was energized by the supply voltage which values were selected from the range of $(0, 2U_N)$; measurements have been carried out using two methods simultaneously. During measurements made by means of electric method, PD signals were detected by 120 seconds for each value of applied supply voltage (time period of data registration demanded to realize calculations made in analysis mode and by means of TEAS program). AE signals were recorded four times for each value of selected supply voltages within time periods of 2 seconds.

Many bars have been tested by the Authors. Measurement results and their analysis, presented in the article, deal with two selected bars (in which PD appeared) marked as:

–bar „D" (coil bar of the generator 120 MW, U_N=13.8 kV),

–bar „M" (coil bar of the generator 200 MW, UN=15.76 kV).

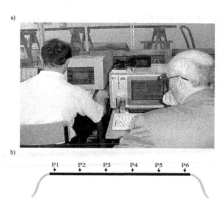

Figure 5. General view of the measuring stand to PD investigation in coil bars of generators with measuring systems DEMA-COMP and TE 571 (a) as well as arrangement of measuring points applied during PD testing by means of AE method in coils bars of generators (b)

U	Q	Diagnosis results received from TEAS program:
kV	nC	Kind of PD source – correctness of diagnose (estimation by probability)
10	3.5	Inclusions near HV electrode (inside dielectric, near surface of the bar) – 0.57
15	3.8	Inclusions near HV electrode (inside dielectric, near surface of the bar) – 0.41 Inclusions near LV electrode (in upper part of dielectric) – 0.21 Inclusions inside dielectric – 0.15
20	2.2	Inclusions near HV electrode (inside dielectric, near surface of the bar) – 0.39
25	2.2	Inclusions near HV electrode (inside dielectric, near surface of the bar) – 0.44
30	2.0	Inclusions near HV electrode (inside dielectric, near surface of the bar) – 0.86

Table 1. Results of analysis of PD phenomena within the bar „D" (U_N=13.8 kV) - electric method

U	Q	Diagnosis results received from TEAS program:
kV	nC	Kind of PD source – correctness of diagnose (estimation by probability)
10	2.2	External disturbances – 0.03
15	3.4	Superposition of inner discharges and corona (own analysis of Authors for lack of a standard in the library of profiles)
20	6.5	Discharge inside dielectric, 1% surface discharge – 0.12
25	70	Corona appeared at many points which dominates inner discharges – 0.21
30	26	Corona appeared at many points which dominates inner discharges – 0.26

Table 2. Results of analysis of PD phenomena within the bar „M" (U_N=15.76 kV) - electric method

6. Results of PD analysis received from electric tests

Results of PD analysis in the bars carried out after measurements made by means of electric method (using system TE 571) are presented in Tables 1 and 2. Two bars are interesting from the point of view of analysis of PD sources. Apparent charges introduced by PD sources in the bar „D" is order of a few or several dozen nanoCulombs. Their value increases as the supply voltage increases. Values of apparent charges introduced by PD sources to the bar „M" are anomalous (70 nC).

7. EA basic properties of AE signals coming from partial discharges in generator coil bars

Exemplary descriptions of AE signals recorded within bars „D" and „M" in the measuring channel with WD sensor are presented in Figs. 1 and 6. All elements of these descriptions have been received using signal filtration by means of pass-band filter of 5. order and signal band of 20 - 500 kHz.

The following bands in the signal spectrum are visible at the diagrams „b", "e" and „f" situated in Figs. 1 and 6: 20 - 40 kHz, 70 - 110 kHz, 120 - 150 kHz, 200 - 240 kHz, 270 - 290 kHz and 450-490 kHz. Analysis of descriptions registered at other measuring points and made for other values of the supply voltage proves representativeness of indicated frequency bands.

Characteristic c), d) and f) from Figs. 1 and 6 show analyzed quantities in dependence on a phase of the supply voltage. Characteristics d) and f) prove periodical character of PD in all cases, evolved by appearance of maximums of the tested quantity, twice during averaging period of the supply voltage.

Characteristics c) of mentioned Figures - this means phase-time diagrams, enable us to analyze values of AE signal amplitude for an established phase in successive periods of the supply voltage. They show two features: greater values appear for phase ranges (at the diagram are visible two „corridors") and phase diagrams of signal amplitudes show fluctuation of these values for successive periods of the supply voltage.

From Fig. 7 results that - for frequencies greater than 150 kHz - frequency characteristic of a measuring channel is flat, therefore all characteristics of AE signals show entirely quantity properties of PD phenomena. Properties of investigated phenomena in the range of frequency from 20 to 150 kHz are „rescaled" by noise of a measuring channel.

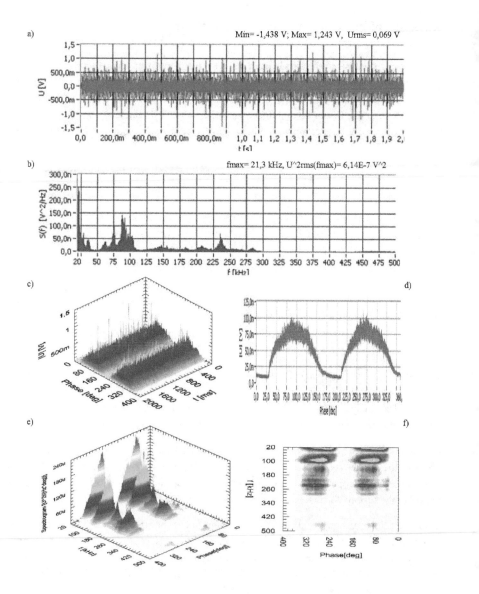

Figure 6. Description of AE signal recorded in the measuring conditions - measurement by means of WD sensor placed at P2 measuring point of „D" bar, the supply voltage of the bar 20 kV, measured value of the apparent charge 2.2 nC: a) impulse (after filtration), b) frequency characteristic, c) phase-time characteristic, d) averaging phase characteristic, e) and f) averaging STFT spectrograms

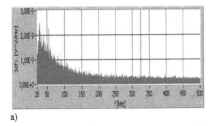 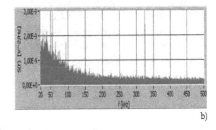

a)   b)

Figure 7. Frequency characteristics of noises in the measuring channel recorded in the following measuring conditions: bar „D", 0 kV, measuring point P1, AE sensor - WD: a) noises before measurements, b) noises after measurements

8. Location of PD sources by means of a method based on advanced degree of AE signals

8.1. Basis of location of PD sources by means of AE method

AE impulses are generated in PD source and propagate in the whole volume of a medium as
AE elastic waves. They are subjected to phenomena connected with propagation of waves and
particularly - dumping during propagation. In a such a way, AE signals which attained a given
measuring point have amplitudes „weighted" by length of propagation path of a signal from
PD source to AE sensor. Signals of less propagation path have more weight. This process
depends also on frequency because AE elastic waves are damped during propagation and
damping is stronger for higher frequencies.

From Fig. 2g results that - even in the frame of one period of the supply voltage – AE signals
coming from many partial discharges reach EA sensor placed at one measuring point.
Registration of AE signals requires multiple assembly of the sensor at chosen measuring points.
In practice, that changes conditions of registration because – despite of repeatable procedure
of mounting of the sensor – there is not certainty that the coupling layer will be stable and
parallel.

From these reasons, even though a tested object should be treated as one-dimensional, Authors
consider traditional methods of location of PD sources as insufficient ones. Instead of traditional approach the new method of location is proposed. Such a method is based on defined
descriptors, calculated for recorded AE signals. In analyzed cases measurements were realized
for each tested bars. That gives a set of 144 recorded AE signals (6 measuring points P1, P2,
P3, P4, P5 and P6; 6 selected values of the supply voltage: 0, 10, 15, 20, 25 and 30 kV; 4 AE signals
recorded at each measuring point for each chosen value of the supply voltage).

The following activities are proceeded: choice of filtration band of recorded signals, filtration
of all signals, calculation of amplitude distributions and AE descriptors.

Now, the procedure is as follows: a) calculation of mean values and standard deviation of AE descriptor for signals recorded at a given measuring point and under determined value of the supply voltage, b) determination of dependencies of AE descriptor values on position of a measuring point for determined value of the supply voltage, c) search of maximums at received curves whose locate PD sources.

The presented way of location of PD sources was named by Authors as the method based on advanced degree of AE signal.

8.2. Location of PD sources in the band of [150,500] kHz by means of AE method

Location of PD sources on the basis of advanced degree of AE signal was begun from the band of 150 – 500 kHz. According to analysis presented at point 7, amplitude-frequency characteristic of the measuring system is plate within this band of frequency, then AE signals are not changed during their recording. Since „forced" damping along propagation path is expected so contribution from the nearest source should be dominant within recorded signals.

Diagrams of ADP descriptor values within Figs. 8 are expressed depending on of position of a measuring point for two tested bars and different values of the supply voltage. Maximums at each curve locate PD sources.

Results of location of PD sources with maximal activity for „D" bar are as follows:

a. when the supply voltages is 10 kV then PD source with maximal activity is situated near measuring point P2,

b. when supply voltages are 15 kV and 20 kV then PD source with maximal activity situated near measuring point P2 is still active, but there is also the second source near measuring point P5,

c. when supply voltages are 25 kV and 30 kV then local maximums remain identical as for 15 kV and 20 kV, but differences between local maximum and local minimum at the curve are considerable smaller (by comparison with curves for supply voltages 15 kV and 20 kV).

Statement of descriptor families for particular supply voltages gives additional information about location of PD sources. AE signals for lower supply voltages are recorded only at measuring points situated nearby PD sources, whereas AE signals for high supply voltages are recorded at all measuring points. In the last case „weighing" of AE signals enables us to locate PD sources as before. Elongation of propagation path of AE signals when the supply voltage increases is caused by differentiation of their power; AE signals recorded under supply voltages 25 kV and 30 kV have the power many times greater than the power of AE signals recorded under 10 kV. Greater amplitude of AE signal enables us to detect AE signals at measuring points situated farther from PD sources.

It is worth noticing that descriptors for repeatedly measured AE signals, which are noises of a measuring path (different bars and different measuring points), are similar values: about 100 contractual units.

Local maximums for the bar „M" appear in the vicinity of measuring point P3. They are distinct for supply voltages 10, 20, 25 and 30 kV. The second maximum appears near measuring point P5 (for supply voltages 10, 15 and 30 kV). From the supply voltage of 15 kV there are additional processes at one or two ends of the bar whose overlap to this picture.

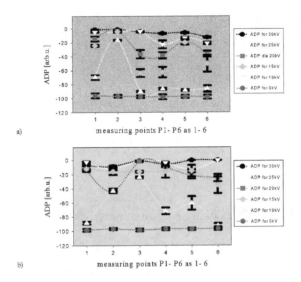

a)

b)

Figure 8. Location of PD sources made by means of method of advanced degree of AE signal (for AE signals registered by WD sensor at measuring points P1-P6, analysis in the band of 150 - 500 kHz) for different values of the supply voltage: a) bar „D", b) bar „M"

8.3. Location of PD sources in the band of [20,60] kHz by means of AE method

Amplitude-frequency characteristic of the measuring system is not flat within selected band of frequencies therefore AE signals are changed during recording. This input, coming from the measuring system, increases monotonically as frequency is decreased; it gives four times growth in spectrum characteristic of density of the power. Additionally (taking into account that damping of elastic waves is greater for higher frequencies) AE elastic waves coming from father distances can be also detected at measuring points within selected bands.

Suitable calculations have been carried out for two tested bars. Diagrams of ADP descriptor values (for signals recorded by R6 sensors) versus the position of a measuring point, for different values of the supply voltage, are presented in Fig. 9.

Location of PD sources within the band of 60 - 20 kHz, resultant from analysis of location of maximums at each curve presented in Fig. 9, gives the following results:

- „D" bar – PD sources are located near the measuring point P2 (under supply voltages of 10, 15, 20, 25 and 30 kV) and P5 (under supply voltages of 20, 25 and 30 kV);

- „M" bar – PD sources are located near the measuring point P3 (appear under all values of supply voltages) and P5 (under supply voltages of 10, 15 and 20 kV), unilateral maximums appear under supply voltages of 25 and 30 kV.

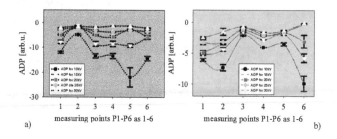

Figure 9. Location of PD sources made by means of the method of advanced degree of AE signal (for AE signals recorded by R6 sensor at measuring points P1-P6, analysis in the band of 20 - 60 kHz) for different values of the supply voltage: a) bar „D", b) bar „M"

9. Location of PD sources using Kohonen network

9.1. Basis for location of PD sources using Kohonen network

Groups of amplitude distributions can be treated as sets of pictures, i.e. input vectors X. In order to describe these sets one should divide them into classes and build pictures representative for particular classes. A good tool for solution of such a task are neuron networks [18-21].

The assigned task imposes the choice of a network which ensures learning of classification without inspection, based on assembly of input data. Lack of information on attachment of input pictures to determined classes, established a priori, shows that searched network has self organization features, i.e. it finds by one-self standards within input data and codes them (in order to find of output). In the stage of selection of the network the following assumption has been made – only one output unity is in active state during learning at a given moment. Output unities compete with themselves in order to be within the incited state and are named unities type of „winner takes all" (WTA).

The above requirements fulfill the networks in which competitive learning without inspection has place [19,21], i.e. self-organized networks where the base is competition between neurons. These networks include input layer and self-organized one. Input layer is defined by dimension of input vector (N). Self-organizing layer contains M neurons with a structure defined during solution of specific problem. In practice, WTA algorithm has been replaced by winner take most (WTM) algorithms in which - besides a winner - neighbouring neurons actualize also their weights (the greater distance from a winner the less change of the value of neuron weights). An example of WTM algorithm is one of Grossberg-Kohonen. Authors have implemented Kohonen neuron network using a set of tools coming from DataEngine V.i. worked up on the base of LabView software. Operation of the network is realized by means of „Kohonen EA" program (written for this purpose) which realizes the following tasks:

–building of Kohonen network and standard pictures for the classes,

–labeling of classes,

–testing of input objects.

Kohonen network is built after introduction of input data (learning data) and after determination of number of features within input vector, number of layers and winning neurons. Input data make a set of input vectors. Single input vector (vector of features) has the following form:

$$\vec{X}^T =[A_1,A_2,...,A_p,B_1,B_2,...,B_q,C_1,C_2,...,C_r,D_1,D_2,...,D_s] \tag{2}$$

where $\vec{A}$ and $\vec{C}$ are amplitude distributions of AE counts and the power of a signal, whereas $\vec{B}$ and $\vec{D}$ are derivatives of $\vec{B}$ and $\vec{D}$ against discrimination threshold.

A single value of vector component X_a^T (single feature) is one of values of one of AE amplitude distributions or their derivatives for a given discrimination threshold U_T. Full definition of an input vector needs determination of parameters p, q, r and s. These parameters are determined during preparation of learning data – by means of „AE amplitude distributions and descriptors" program. Input vector includes amplitude distributions of a signal; input data describe signal families. Up to the present, an assumption has been put during analyses: contribution of each from amplitude distributions to a final result is the same. This assumption is realized by means of the same values of parameters p, q, r and s as well as by normalization of independent groups of particular amplitude distributions.

Implemented Kohonen network is built by two layers – input one and Kohonen layer. Number of neurons in input layer is a number of features characterized a given problem ($p+q+r+s$). Kohonen layer is many-dimensional table of neurons – number of dimensions 1, 2 or 3 is optional (number of neurons in Kohonen layer was established experimentally). Adaptation of weights is realized according to Grossberg-Kohonen algorithm; learning constant and neighbouring ray are changed during learning during successive input vectors are analyzed. This dynamic of the network aims at improvement of activity and organization of neurons during learning process. Such a dynamic of neuron network is written as an dependence of quantities $\vec{W}$, η and G versus t (time):

$$\Delta\vec{W}(t+1) = \eta(t)G(t)[\vec{X}-\vec{W}] \tag{3}$$

Final vector of weights of a given neuron reflects values of features of a vector representative for a given class; result describes ability to fragmentation of a set of input pictures to separable classes and creation representative standard pictures for these classes.

Kohonen network may realize the task consisting in assignment of input vectors of particular classes. Input vectors can be learning data for realized network or any input vectors with identical structure of features. Input vectors are built by means of „AE amplitude distributions and AE descriptors" program. They are the form which is recognized by „AE Kohonen" program. Choice of features of input vector is essential problem for results obtained by built Kohonen network. Authors chose amplitude distributions ADC and ADP as well as derivative of these descriptions (against discrimination threshold), assimilating input data to problems of Newton dynamics. Additionally, concerning about discernment of pictures by Kohonen network, amplitude distributions are prepared in logarithmic scale. Owing to that, input pictures distinguish exponential character of many phenomena. It is worth addition that such a form of input data (which takes into account physical aspects of researched phenomenon) leads to a proper classification. „AE Kohonen" program normalizes input vectors (normalization is made independently within one distribution kind because it gives the same contribution of each distribution into realized input vector), classifies, builds winning neurons and enables us to classify input vectors.

9.2. Location of PD sources in the band of [150,500] kHz using Kohonen network

Results of classification of 144 input vectors (for each bar) made by Kohonen network, built for 10 winning neurons have been assembled to subgroups included input vectors for particular values of the supply voltage (0, 10, 15, 20, 25 and 30 kV). Each subgroup contains 24 series describing input vectors for AE signals, recorded at particular measuring points (4 measuring series for each measuring point - P1, P2, P3, P4, P5 and P6 successively). Assembled location results are presented in Fig. 10.

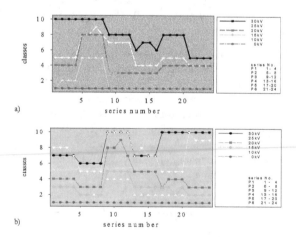

Figure 10. Classification results of input vectors (for AE signals recorded by WD sensor at measuring points P1-P6, analysis in the band of 150 - 500 kHz) by Kohonen network for different values of the supply voltage: a) bar „D", b) bar „M" (maximum within a subgroup locates PD source with maximum activity)

Location is made within subgroups (for particular supply voltages) by determination of the measuring point where local maximum appears. Higher class given by the network correspond with higher advanced degree of AE signal.

Results of location of PD sources for both bars by means of Kohonen network are as follows:

a. PD sources within „D" are located near measuring point P2 (for each values of the supply voltage) and near P5 (for supply voltages of 15, 20, 25 and 30 kV),

b. PD sources within „M" are located near measuring point P3 (for each values of the supply voltage) and near P5 (for the supply voltage of 20 kV), but from beginning of 15 kV additional processes appear at one or two ends of the bar (they overlap on this picture).

It is worth also noticing the following facts:

1. Kohonen network gives the lowest class (class 1) to input vectors for noises of a measuring channel,

2. Kohonen network gives classes which differ most of two ones to particular input vectors built for signals recorded at one point and under one supply voltage (it may recognize that deformation processes are stable),

3. there is conformability between location made by means of the method of descriptors and when Kohonen network is applied (Figs. 7 and 8).

10. Location of PD sources — Recapitulation

There are two PD sources within bar „D" near measuring points P2 and P5 whose were named as Z1 and Z2 respectively.

There are two PD sources within bar „M" near measuring points P3 and P5 whose were named as Z3 and Z4 respectively as well as two sources at ends of the bar named as Z5 and Z6.

Z1 and Z3 sources are active under supply voltages of 10, 15, 20, 25 and 30 kV. Z2 source is active beginning from supply voltages of 10 or 15 kV. Z5 and Z6 sources are active under higher values of the supply voltage 25 and 30 kV.

Results of location of PD sources coming from the method of descriptors and Kohonen network are identical in practice.

It is worth noticing the following information, included in Figs. 8 and 9:

a. signals generated by Z1 source in the band of 150 - 500 kHz may be detected up to distance of 1 m (for lowered bands the distance is longer),

b. AE signals are recorded within the band of 20 - 60 kHz at all measuring points even under the supply voltage of 10 kV,

c. there are not different AE sources after changing of frequency bands.

Conclusions a) and b) result from physics of elastic waves. The conclusion c) proves that bars are „grateful" research material, in which there are not other significant acoustic phenomena masked of PD like, for example, in oil power transformers.

11. Description of AE impulses radiated by PD sources (band of [150, 500] kHz)

Description of AE signals coming from PD sources, named as Z1, Z2, Z3 and Z6, is presented in Figs. 11 - 14. Characteristics of these selected AE signals are beginning of data base describing AE signals generated by PD sources within coil bars of generators.

Properties of AE signals coming from particular sources are as follows:

- Z1 source – averaging phase-time characteristic is characterized by: trapezoid shape, asymmetry of amplitude and shape in both half of the period, asymmetry of amplitudes of averaging STFT spectrogram, frequency main bands of 230 – 250 kHz (main bands) and remaining bands of 280 – 290 kHz;

- Z2 source – averaging phase-time characteristic is characterized by: shape of Gauss curve, symmetry of amplitude and shape in both half of the period, symmetry of amplitudes of averaging STFT spectrogram, frequency main bands of 230 – 240 kHz (main bands) and remaining bands of 280 – 290 kHz;

- Z3 source – averaging phase-time characteristic is characterized by: triangle-trapezoid shape, asymmetry of amplitude and shape in both half of the period, symmetry of ampli-tudes of averaging STFT spectrogram, frequency main bands of 230 – 250 kHz and remaining bands of 280 – 290 kHz;

- Z6 source – averaging phase-time characteristic is characterized by: triangle shape, sym-metry of amplitude and shape in both half of the period, symmetry of amplitudes of averaging STFT spectrogram, main frequency bands of 230 kHz – 245 kHz and remaining bands of 280 – 290 kHz.

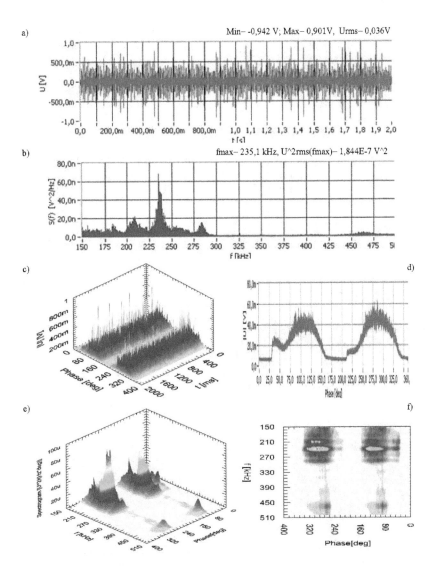

Figure 11. Z1 source: a) impulse (after filtration), b) frequency characteristic, c) phase-time characteristic, d) averaging phase characteristic, e) and f) averaging STFT spectrograms recorded in measuring conditions: measurement by means of WD sensor placed at P2 measuring point of „D" bar, the supply voltage of the bar 11.8 kV, measured value of the apparent charge 3.8 nC

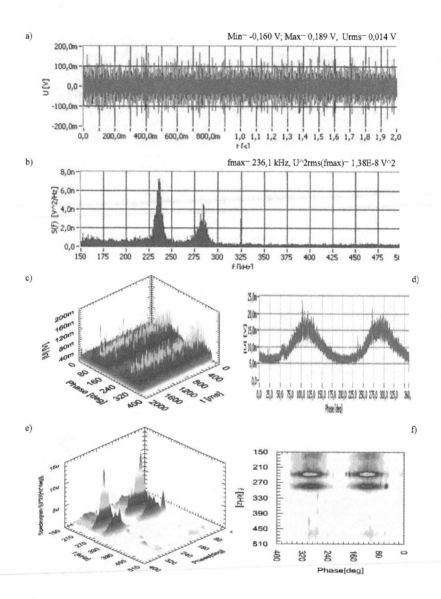

Figure 12. Z2 source: a) impulse (after filtration), b) frequency characteristic, c) phase-time characteristic, d) averaging phase characteristic, e) and f) averaging STFT spectrograms recorded in measuring conditions: measurement by means of WD sensor placed at P5 measuring point of „D" bar, the supply voltage of the bar 20.5 kV, measured value of the apparent charge 2.2 nC

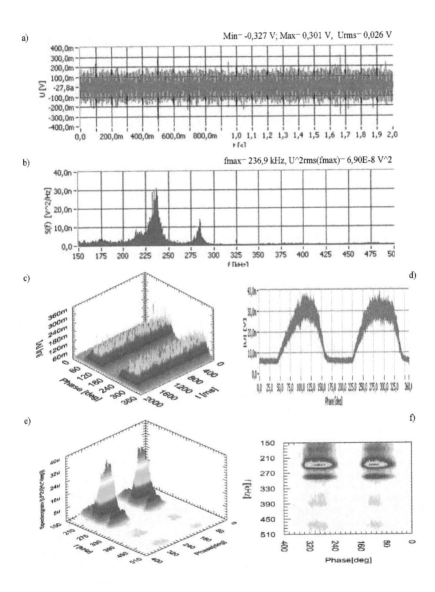

Figure 13. Z3 source: a) description of AE signal, b) frequency characteristic, c) phase-time characteristic, d) averaging phase characteristic, e) and f) averaging STFT spectrograms recorded in measuring conditions: measurement by means of WD sensor placed at P3 measuring point of „M" bar, the supply voltage of the bar 15.5 kV, measured value of the apparent charge 3.4 nC

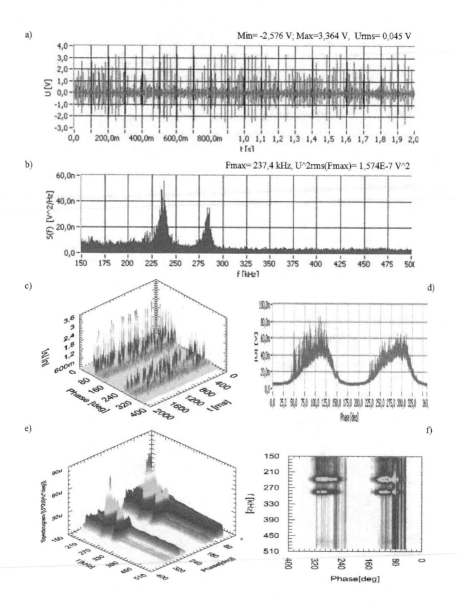

Figure 14. Z6 source: a) description of AE signal, b) frequency characteristic, c) phase-time characteristic, d) averaging phase characteristic, e) and f) averaging STFT spectrograms recorded in measuring conditions: measurement by means of WD sensor placed at P6 measuring point of „M" bar, the supply voltage of the bar 31 kV, measured value of the apparent charge 26 nC

12. Cumulative analysis of PD testing results made by means of joint electric-acoustic methodology

Results of analyses concerning testing of PD within „D" and „M" bar, received simultaneously from electric and AE method, are stated in Tables 3 and 4. The statement contains supply voltages and the following measured or calculated quantities for signals recorded under particular supply voltages: apparent charge, ADP descriptors for AE signal which gives maximum within the suitable group of AE signals (after analysis within bands of 150 – 500 kHz and 20 – 60 kHz) and properties of PD sources determine independently by means of electric and acoustic method. There are properties: kind of PD determined by means of expert diagnostic program TEAS (electric method) and location of PD sources (AE method). Such a statement enables us to obtain more complete information on the kind and the place in which partial discharges appear.

		Electric method	AE method		
U	Q	Diagnosis results received from TEAS program:	ADP within bands of:		Location of sources
kV	nC	Kind of PD source – correctness of diagnose (estimation by probability)	[150,500] kHz	[20,60] kHz	
10	3.5	Inclusions near HV electrode (inside dielectric, near surface of the bar) – 0.57	-16.3	-4.9	Z1 source – near P2
15	3.8	Inclusions near HV electrode (inside dielectric, near surface of the bar) – 0.41 Inclusions near LV electrode (in upper part of dielectric) – 0.21 Inclusions inside dielectric – 0.15	-4.2	-1.2	Z1 source – near P2 Z2 source – near P5
20	2.2	Inclusions near HV electrode (inside dielectric, near surface of the bar) – 0.39	-3.3	-2.2	Z1 source – near P2 Z2 source – near P5
25	2.2	Inclusions near HV electrode (inside dielectric, near surface of the bar) – 0.44	-4.0	-2.7	Z1 source – near P2 Z2 source – near P5
30	2.0	Inclusions near HV electrode (inside dielectric, near surface of the bar) – 0.86	-1.3	-1.6	Z1 source – near P2 Z2 source – near P5

Table 3. Statement of results of PD analysis made by means of electric-acoustic methodology for „D" bar (U_N =13.8 kV)

The source of the most intensive partial discharges appears within „D" bar near measuring point P2. This source is created by inclusions near HV electrode (inside dielectric, near surface of the bar). Ignition of partial discharges at point P2 takes place already under the supply voltage of 7 kV (about 52% U_N). This source is created by inclusions near LV electrode. The most compose description of PD, given by expert diagnostic program TEAS (for the supply voltage 15 kV), corresponds with activity of Z1 source and growth of activity of Z2 source. Growth of apparent charge value is caused by properties of PD source which is located near point P2. Maximal value of ADP descriptor and maximal value of apparent charge was registered for the band of 20 – 60 kHz under the supply voltage of 15 kV.

Electric method			AE method		
U	Q	Diagnosis results received from TEAS program: Kind of PD source – correctness of diagnose (estimation by probability)	ADP within bands of:		Location of sources
kV	nC		[150,500] kHz	[20,60] kHz	
10	2.2	External disturbances – 0.03	-24.0	-2.1	Z3 source – near P3 Z4 source – near P5
15	3.4	Superposition of inner discharges and corona (own analysis of Authors for lack of a standard in the library of profiles)	-15.8	-1.6	Z3 source – near P3 Z4 source – near P5
20	6.5	Discharge inside dielectric, 1% surface discharge – 0.12	-1.4	-1.2	Z3 source – near P3 Z4 source – near P5
25	70	Corona appeared at many points which dominates inner discharges – 0.21	-0.4	-1.0	Z3 source – near P3 Z4 source – near P5 Z5,Z6 sources – near ends
30	26	Corona appeared at many points which dominates inner discharges – 0.26	-1.0	-0.7	Z3 source – near P3 Z4 source – near P5 Z5,Z6 sources – near ends

Table 4. Statement of results of PD analysis made by means of electric-acoustic methodology for „M" bar (U_N =13.8 kV)

The source of the most intensive partial discharges within „M" bar appears near measuring point P3. It is caused by inner discharges. Additionally, the source within area of measuring points P5 and P6 is active for supply voltages 25 and 30 kV. There is also a source near measuring point P5 within the band of 20 – 60 kHz. Acoustic method shows weak sensitivity for many-point corona discharge given growth of apparent charge up to value of 70 nC.

13. Recapitulation

The original method, worked out to analyze of AE signals at basic and advanced level, is presented. The basic analysis is made in domains of time, frequency and time-frequency, whereas advanced analysis describes properties of AE signals in domain of threshold.

The results of basic analysis are as follows:

–the signal after filtration with its minimal, maximal and RMS values (the band pass filter of 5. order is applied to filtration which band is given as a frequency range at the frequency characteristic),

–spectral power density as frequency characteristic of the signal with the frequency for main maximum and spectrum value for this frequency,

–phase-time characteristic,

–averaging phase characteristic,

–three-dimensional STFT spectrogram,

–three-dimensional STFT spectrogram dropped to a phase-frequency plane.

These quantities are calculated for AE signals recorded during 100 periods of the supply voltage and describes properties of AE signal for „averaging" period of the supply voltage. They define frequency of bands dominant within AE signals and describe random character of AE signals appearing in analyzed phenomena.

Results of advanced analysis are distributions of counting rate and power of the signal in function of discrimination threshold as well as ADC and ADP descriptors which describe quantitatively AE signals named as advanced degree of recorded AE signals. Descriptors are a base to locate PD sources by means of advanced degree of AE signals.

Investigations of partial discharges within generator coil bars, realized as simultaneous measurements made by means of electric and acoustic method. Electric method was applied to determine apparent charge, introduced by active PD sources, and kind of recorded partial discharges (by means of TEAS program). Analysis of test results is presented for two chosen bars, designed as „D" (bar of the coil of the generator 120 MW, U_N=13.8 kV) and „M" (bar of the coil of the generator 200 MW, U_N=15.76 kV). The both bars are interesting from the point of vue of analyze of PD sources. In the case of „D" bar, PD sources introduce apparent charges whose value is at the level of several nC; this value diminues when the supply voltage increases. Values of apparent charges introduced by PD sources into „M" bar reached suprising anomalous great value (70 nC).

AE measurements were made at six measuring points of each tested bar. Investigation results obtained from AE method determine the following frequency bands, dominant in AE signals: 20 - 40 kHz, 70 - 110 kHz, 120 - 150 kHz, 200 - 240 kHz, 270 - 290 kHz and 450-490 kHz. ADC and ADP descriptors calculated for recorded signals order theses signals according their advanced degree. They are a base for location of AE sources by means of the original method of advanced degree of AE signals.

In result of analysis of AE signals within the band of [150,500] kHz such a location od PD sources for different values of the supply voltage have been made; six PD sources were located and results of basic analysis for these sources were presented.

Obtained results were proved by location resultant from application of Kohonen network.

AE signals recorded within the band [20,60] kHz were analyzed additionally. Analysis of AE signals in different frequency bands showed the same location of PD sources and proved changes of AE signals during propagation.

The cumulative analysis of PD test results made by means of complex electric-accoustic methodology enables us to obtain more complete information about the kind and the place of occurrence of partial discharges.

Author details

Franciszek Witos[1] and Zbigniew Gacek[2]

*Address all correspondence to: franciszek.witos@polsl.pl

1 Department of Optoelectronics, Silesian University of Technology, Gliwice, Poland

2 Institute of Power Systems & Control, Silesian University of Technology, Gliwice, Poland

References

[1] Bartnikas, P. *PDs their mechanism, detection and measurement,* IEEE Trans. on Dielectrics and Electrical Insulation, (2002). , 9(5), 763-808.

[2] Lundgaard, L. E. *PD- part Xii: acoustic PD detection- fundamental considerations,*IEEE EI Magazine, (1992). , 8(4), 25-31.

[3] Lundgaard, L. E. *PD-part: Xii acoustic PD detection- practical application*IEEE EI Magazine, (1992). , 8(5), 34-43.

[4] Witos, F, Gacek, Z, & Opilski, A. The new AE descriptor for modeled sources of PDs, Archives of Acoustic, (2002). , 27(1), 65-77.

[5] Witos, F, & Gacek, Z. *In search of AE descriptors correlated with apparent electric charge*, ISH- XIIIth Int Symposium on High Voltage Engineering, Netherlands (2003). Smit (ed.) 2003 Milpress, Rotterdam

[6] Boczar, T, Borucki, S, Cichon, A, & Zmarzly, D. Application possibilities of artificial neural networks for recognizing partial discharges measured by the acoustic emission method, IEEE Trans. on Dielectrics and Electrical Insulation, (2009). , 16(3), 214-223.

[7] Witos, F, & Gacek, Z. Application of the calibrated AE to investigate properties of AE signals coming from PD sources modeled in laminar systems, Journal de Physique IV, (2005). , 129, 173-177.

[8] Witos, F, & Gacek, Z. *Application of the joint electro-acoustic method for PD investigation within a power transformer,* European Physical Journal ST, (2008). , 154

[9] LabVIEW™ and LabWindows™/CVI™*Signal Proces. Toolset User Manual*, National Instruments, (2005).

[10] Dabrowski, M. Construction of electrical machines, WNT, Warsaw, Poland (1997). in Polish).

[11] Zondervan, J. P, Gulski, E, & Smit, J. J. *Fundamental aspects of PD pattern of on-line measurements of turbogenerators,* IEEE Trans. on Dielectric and EI, (2000). , 7(1), 59-70.

[12] Witos, F, & Gacek, Z. *Investigations of PDs in generator coil bars by means of AE: acoustic images and location,* CIGRE 39th Int. Session, Paris (2002). (11-101), 11-101.

[13] Kaneko, T. et all: *Characterization of on-line PD in stator winding on starting hydrogenerator using AE detection method,*ISH- XIIIth Int Symposium on High Voltage Engineering, Netherlands (2003). Smit (ed.) 2003 Milpress, Rotterdam.

[14] Witos, F, Gacek, Z, & Opilski, Z. *Testing of Partial Discharges in Generator Coil Bars with the Help of Calibrated Acoustic Emission Method,*Acta Physica Polonica A, (2008). , 114(6-A), 249-258.

[15] Kaneko, T. et all: Characteristics of on-line and off-line partial discharge on hydrogenerator stator windings using acoustic emission detection techniques,, (2005). Proceedings of 2005 International Symposium on Electrical Insulating Materials (ISEIM 2005),5-9 June 2005

[16] Partial Discharge Detector Type TE 571Operating Manual, (2005). , 2

[17] Physical Acoustics Corporation: . *www.pacndt.com.*

[18] Tadeusiewicz, R. *Neural Networks*, Academic Of. Ed. RM, Warsaw, Poland (1993). in Polish).

[19] Hertz, J, Krogh, A, & Palmer, R. G. *Introduction to the theory of neural computation,* WNT, Warsaw, Poland (1995). in Polish).

[20] Zurada, J, Barski, M, & Jedruch, W. *Artificial neural networks,* PWN, Warsaw, Poland (1996). in Polish).

[21] Ossowski, S. *Neural networks for information processing,* Of. Ed. Pol. Warsaw, Warsaw, Poland (2000). in Polish).

Chapter 8

Application of Acoustic Emission for Quality Evaluation of Fruits and Vegetables

Artur Zdunek

Additional information is available at the end of the chapter

1. Introduction

Food crushing sound is one of the main factors used for food quality evaluation. Crispness and crunchiness are attributes of high quality product and are usually pointed on the top of a list of consumer preferences. However, the meanings of crispness and crunchiness are still imprecise. Its perception varies from country to country and from individual to individual. Despite of this there is a general consensus that crispy and crunchy sensation is related to fracture properties. Crispy product is mechanically brittle, firm and acoustically noisy as a result of large number of small fractures. Crunchiness is probably related to events (fractures) occurring on subsequent layers in a cell structure what gives the sense of extension of sound duration in time.

In spite of sensory and subjective nature of food quality evaluation by human senses, a big effort is put for objective sound properties analysis during biting and chewing and for developing instrumental methods for human independent food evaluation. The first instrumental analysis of sound was published by Drake in 1963, who found that crisper products emit louder sound and an average amplitude of successive bursts during mastication decreases [1]. Then, several authors used different sound descriptors for judging a chewing sound, as the number of sound burst in a bite n, the mean amplitude of the burst A or the products of these values nA or $nA/sound\ duration$ [1, 2, 3]. The first hypothesis was that the sense of crispness is an auditory phenomena, i.e. is the air-conducted sound. However, work done by Christensen and Vickers in 1981 showed that crispness may be a vibratory phenomena, i.e. is the bone-conducted sound [4].

Most of studies on crispness and crunchiness concern dry food products, like cakes, chips, etc.. However, this problem has been found as important also for fruits and vegetables called as wet food products. In 2002, presumably for the first time, Fillion and Kilcast stated

that crispness and crunchiness are very complex concept containing sound, fracture characteristic, density and geometry of fruit and vegetables [5]. They found that crispy wet food
would refer to a light and thin texture producing a sharp clean break with a high-pitch
sound mainly during the first bite with the front teeth. Crunchy wet food would be hard
and has a dense texture producing loud, low-pitch sound that occurs over successive chews.

Many instrumental methods have been applied for crispness and crunchiness evaluation of
fruits and vegetables. Due to the fact that mastication is a highly destructive process, mechanical tests are the most popular to simulate the biting. Results of such tests, like texture profile
analysis, compression, tension, twist or three-point bending, show correlation with properties
of a material thus can be also used for its texture evaluation. One of the simplest is a puncture
test where probe is pushed into tissue and a maximum force is used as a firmness value.

As it was obtained by Christensen and Vickers [4] crispness may by the bone-conducted
phenomena. Therefore, the acoustic emission (AE) method where a sensor is in a contact
with material investigated is promising tool for food properties evaluation. In general, the
acoustic emission is monitored during deformation of a material to provide information on
cracking and internal friction of material pieces by analysis of AE descriptors like: amplitude, frequency, energy, counts, events, etc..

2. Tissue model and source of AE in fruit and vegetables

The largest volume of fruit and vegetable tissue is taken by parenchymatous cells therefore
this part of fruit is particularly often studied, also from the reason that it is relatively easy to
cut a sample for testing. A simplified model of parenchyma tissue, which considers the most
important mechanical actors, is shown in Fig. 1. The mechanical model is built of cells which
are fluid filled and walls which are elastic-like. Cell walls are made of polysaccharides: cellulose fibrils network embedded in a matrix of pectins and hemicelluloses. Cells adhere to
each other through middle lamellas which are made of amorphous pectins. Tissue structure
also contains intercellular spaces, which for some fruits, like apple, can even take 25%. It is
generally agreed that cell walls have elastic properties whereas pectins in the middle lamella
are plastic-like. External forces which cause deformation of such structure increase a pressure inside the cells and tension in the cell walls. Simultaneously, shearing forces between
cells increase. Thus, two failure modes are possible: cell wall rupturing and cell-cell debonding when strength of cell walls or/and intercellular adhesion is overcome, respectively.
These two processes can be the sources of acoustic emission in the case of cellular plants.
However, acoustic emission from cell-cell debonding due to plastic character is less likely
compared to sudden rupturing of elastic cell walls.

Studying of cracking process of plant tissue is thus indeed important for understanding of
quality of fruits and vegetables. When tissue cracks between cells, for example for fruit and
veggie which have been stored too long, the material may show a mealy character whereas
the fresh one, just after picking up, cracking through cell walls reveals juicy and crispy properties which are usually desired by consumers. Mechanical strength of plant tissue at micro-

structure level is also important not only from the point of view the sensory properties. For example, microcracking is important for blackspot bruising of potato which starts enzymatic browning of the tissue under the skin.

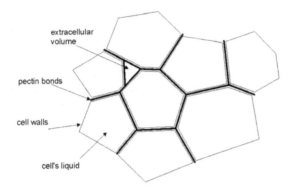

Figure 1. A simplified mechanical model of parenchyma tissue of fruits and vegetables

3. Acoustic emission (AE) for evaluation of the onset of plant tissue cracking

As it is for other solid materials, acoustic emission has been found as a very useful method for monitoring of cracking of plant tissue under external loading. AE has been applied for this group of materials for the first time in the late 90's [6]. The first attempt was aimed on observation of the AE signal from damaged sample of potato tissue. Figure 2 presents scheme of the first apparatus used. A one-column and low noise testing machine was used for studying the mechanical properties and forces that participate in the process of plant tissue cracking. In that work a wide-band piezoelectric sensor was used for the recording of the acoustic emission signal with high-sensitivity in the frequency range from 25 kHz to 1 MHz. Due to a small size of the samples which are usually used in experiments with plants and relatively large deformations which can cause friction between sensor and sample, fixing the AE sensor directly on the sample was impossible. This problem was solved by fixing the sensor to the jaw of the testing machine, like it is shown in the Fig. 2. Since the AE signal passes from the material with lower density and enters into the material with higher density at the border between the sample and the jaw (sample of tissue – steel), sensitivity of measurement is sufficient to record even small AE events. In order to eliminate any friction and improvement of sound conductivity, silicon grease was applied on each boundary on the way of elastic waves from sample to sensor. A set consisted of a pre-amplifier (40dB) with a high-pass filter (25 kHz) and a low-noise amplifier with adjustable gain was used for signal conditioning. The set was supplemented with a high speed transducer card A/D that allowed for the recording of counts, events and energy in time intervals from 0.001 to 1 second or fast sampling with 2.5MHz short samples 0.25 s long.

The most useful method of analysis of AE signal bases on the transformation of the time signals to the form of descriptors recorded in time intervals. If a certain threshold is established for the amplitude of the received signal, called a discrimination threshold, then every time the amplitude goes above this signal is recorded as one count. Groups of the AE signal with the characteristics shape of a damped sinusoid curve are called events (Fig. 3). Instead of analysis the shape of event, it is possible to define an AE event as a group of counts recorded in consecutive samples. The number of counts and the number of events recorded in time gates are called count rate and event rate. Registered AE signal, presented in Fig. 3 in amplitude – time coordinates can be also characterized by AE energy E. Assuming that a signal event of duration t and of peak amplitude V of an event, then energy of each event can be evaluated as:

$$E = 0.5V^2t \tag{1}$$

Besides the parameters mentioned above, other parameters based on the transformations of time or spectrum of the AE signal could be also used. Detailed definitions and descriptions of the AE signal descriptors can be found in literature [7]. The system presented in Fig. 2 also allowed for simultaneous measuring mechanical and acoustical properties. For example, stress and AE counts as a function of strain could be recorded together as it is shown in Fig. 4.

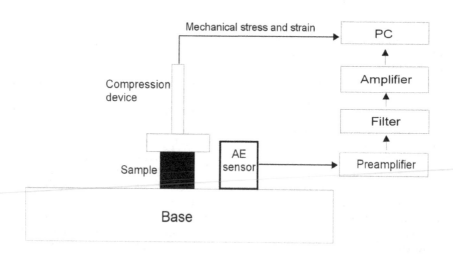

Figure 2. Scheme of the first apparatus used for acoustic emission recording from deformed plant tissue (based on the work of Zdunek and Konstankiewicz [6]). The EA 100 was the analyser which allowed both recording samples with 2.5MHz and conversion of the signal to AE descriptors

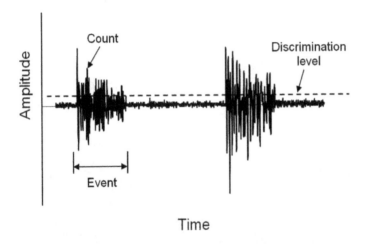

Figure 3. The method of determination of AE descriptors: counts and events from time-amplitude signal. The discrimination level is found experimentally to avoid external noises, for example from the loading device

In Fig. 4 it is easy to notice that for a decrease in the slope of the stress-strain curve (bioyeld and rupture points in this case), a high value of AE counts was observed. The highest values, however, appear at the moment of sudden rupture. Macro-cracks of the samples are clearly visible on the cross-sections of the sample after rupture, and sometimes are even audible to human ears. Before rupture, presumably some cracks also appear, particularly in the region close to bioyield, however it is difficult to detect them visually. The acoustic emission signal shown in Fig. 4 unambiguously proves that bioyield point and rupture could be assigned to tissue cracking, however maybe at different scales. Moreover, a long before bioyeld, AE signal has been detected too, although with significantly lower number of counts. In this region of deformation no noticeable decrease in the slope of the stress-strain curve was observed. Generally, the AE counts before bioyield is more irregular and have lower values in comparison to acoustic signal after bioyield point. It is believed that microcracking is developing gradually due to heterogeneous structure of the plant tissue even before it could be noted from force-deformation curve. This is particularly important because even a small crack of tissue, for example damage of intercellular plasmalemma, could start irreversible biochemical processes which decay quality of the material or affect its function.

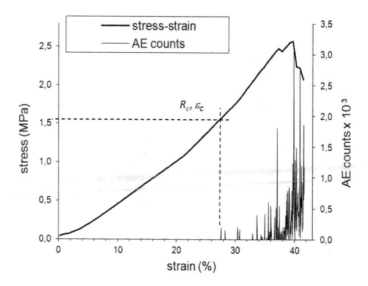

Figure 4. Examples of simultaneous recording of stress, strain and AE counts for potato tuber tissue. Bioyield point is visible as the short drop down of the stress-strain curve, rupture is visible as major final fall down of the stress, and the critical point as the onset of the acoustic signal (AE counts). The critical stress (R_c) and critical strain (ε_c) define the critical point (result obtained by the author)

In the first paper on application of AE for potato tissue, new mechanical parameters have been proposed. Critical stress (R_c) and critical strain (ε_c) have been defined as the mechanical conditions at the onset of acoustic emission. In further studies critical stress and critical strain was analysed under different conditions of mechanical test (Fig. 5) and samples itself (Fig. 6).

Fig. 5 presents how the critical stress and critical strain change with strain rate of two potato cultivars (*Solanum tuberosum* cv. Danusia and Kuba). An increase in the strain rate decreases exponentially both parameters. From microscopic point of view, deformation of plant tissue causes changes in the cell shape. Since initially cells of parenchyma tend to have rounded shape due to incompressibility of the intracellular fluid, the ratio of cells surface to cells volume increases. This means that cell walls are generally stretched during deformation. The tension force in the walls is a function of strain rate and wall permeability. In a simplified model, low strain rate has an effect similar to that of high permeability in the model. At a relatively high strain rate, a seepage of the intracellular fluid through the walls is limited and leads to a higher tensions at the same cell deformation. When the strain rate is low, the intracellular fluid has relatively more time to flow out of the cells, and this produces smaller increases of the tensile forces in the walls. Thus, in this case the strength limit of the cell wall can be reached at higher cell deformation and higher external forces. For relatively slow cell deformation, the cell can even be completely compressed without wall rupture. This explains the pronounced increase of the critical values at very slow rates (Fig. 5).

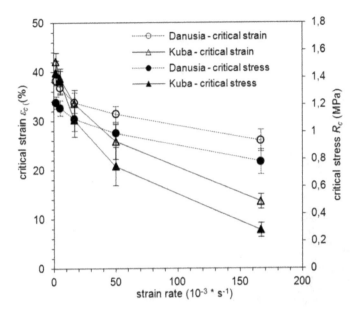

Figure 5. Critical stress and critical strain obtained as the onset of AE during compression of two potato cultivars 'Danusia' and 'Kuba' with different strain rates (result obtained by the author)

The relations between critical stress, critical strain, and osmolality of mannitol solutions in which the samples were hydrated or dehydrated are shown in Fig. 6. Higher osmolality of the mannitol solutions corresponds with lower turgor of the tissue reached after 24h treatment. A strong influence of tissue turgor on critical stress and failure stress was observed. Both critical stress and failure stress increase in a linear manner when turgor decrease (direction of turgor change is shown in Fig. 6). The turgor effect can be interpreted in terms of a model of a single cell. Before deformation, higher turgor causes larger preliminary tension in the cell wall. Thus, the additional cell deformation or the additional external force necessary for wall rupture are lower.

Application of the acoustic emission method has proven that micro-cracking of tissue starts significantly earlier than it can be observed on the stress-strain curve. However, no correlation between the critical values and the failure values of samples tested under the same conditions (the same strain rate or turgor) has been observed [8]. This means that observation of the critical values does not allow prediction of the bioyielding conditions for example. This is presumably result of the fact that critical point and the bioyield point are different stages of cracking. Between them cracking is developing, from the first local micro-cracks to large macro-cracks. This propagation mat be very chaotic and accidental due to heterogeneous microstructure of a tissue.

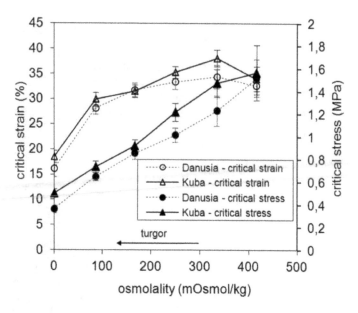

Figure 6. Critical stress and critical strain obtained as the onset of AE during compression of two potato cultivars 'Danusia' and 'Kuba' dehydrated and hydrated in different mannitol solutions (result obtained by the author)

4. Acoustic emission and different mechanical tests

4.1. Puncture test

Application of acoustic emission is possible in any mechanical test which are used commonly for plants. The key issue is to apply AE sensor to the sample which in the case of plants is usually largely deformable. Solution presented previously uses indirect attachment through solid body. This solution was proven to be very effective in various mechanical tests. Sensors of AE could be placed inside device for mechanical tests, exactly in the probe for material deformation. Such device for puncture test is presented in Fig. 7. Here, acoustic emission during the puncture test is caused and recorded by head with two sensors placed inside. The head consists two parts. Top part is made of ertacetal and the bottom part is made of duraluminium which effectively conducts elastic waves. The application of two different material was intended to limit eventual disturbances from mechanical system. They are screwed to each other. Acoustic emission sensors are glued (or it can be screwed also) to the top surface of the metal part. In the system presented in Fig. 7, one sensor works in audible range 1-16kHz (SA), whereas the second sensor has maximum sensitivity in ultrasound range 25-100kHz (SU) to cover as wide as possible frequency region. The sensors are connected to individual amplifiers with adjustable amplifying. The signal is filtered in the range

1 kHz -20 kHz for lower band and 10kHz-900 kHz for higher band. Next, the analogue signals are converted into digital one by A/D boards. Sampling rates per channel: 44 000 and 150 000 samples per second are more than double of the frequency range of the sensors used. The second channel of each card is used for recording an analogue signal of force delivered from universal testing machine to synchronize both acoustic and mechanical signals.

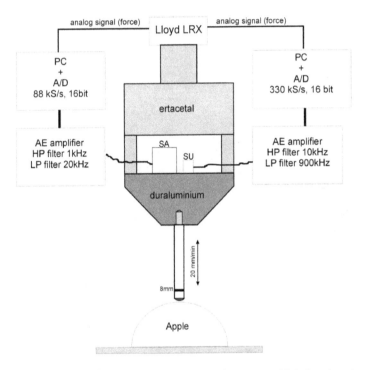

Figure 7. Scheme of the system for recording of acoustic emission from punctured fruit. Two channels were used: 1-16kHz and 20-75 kHz. Puncturing was performed with Lloyd LRX device. SA is the sensor for audible frequencies, SU is the sensor for ultrasound frequencies. Dimensions of the puncture probe are exemplary (scheme by the author)

In Fig. 8, typical profiles of acoustic emission counts recorded during puncturing of apple flesh are shown. In the case of apple puncturing, the AE signal starts just from the moments of touching puncture probe to tissue. The number of counts increases progressively up to a moment when force-deformation curve yields. At this moment the whole curved part of the probe is in a contact with the tissue. When the probe goes deeper into apple tissue the acoustic activity decreases. This could be result of damping of acoustic waves by surrounding tissue and already damaged tissue layers under the probe. In many studies, softening of apples during ripening and storage has been reflected in a lower penetration force (lowering firmness). The integrative use of contact AE and the puncture test showed that major acoustic signals are observed together with drops of force. The coincidence was interpreted as an energy release in the form of sound as a result of material fracturing. In the case of plant tissues, AE signal comes mainly from rupture of the cell wall because of its somewhat elastic properties, whereas the middle lamella due to plastic properties rather do not generate sound. This hypothesis is supported by analysis of AE during ripening of apples, which will be discussed later on in this chapter.

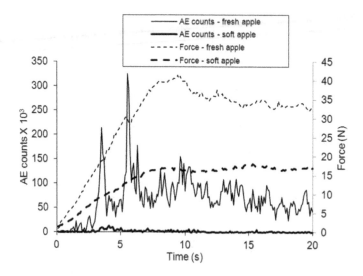

Figure 8. AE counts and force recorded during puncturing of fresh (1 day of shelf life) and stored (10 days of shelf life) apples (result obtained by the author)

In Fig. 9, spectrum of the signal is presented from two frequency ranges in a form of "acustograms". Colors in the acustograms represent a power of the signal in time-frequency coordinates. A few dominant frequencies can be found: 5.5 kHz, 9.5 kHz,15 kHz, 32 kHz, 44 kHz and 56 kHz. They constantly appear during puncturing. Precise analysis showed that they are also characteristic for the system used because no significant changes were found with properties material used. The only one change observed with change of properties of the material was an overall change in amplitude that occurred uniformly for all bands. Additionally, Fig. 10 presents relation between AE energy in 1-16 kHz and 20-75 kHz obtained for a large set of apples in puncture test. It is shown that the relation is very linear and in the case of this material, investigation in higher band does not provide any additional information.

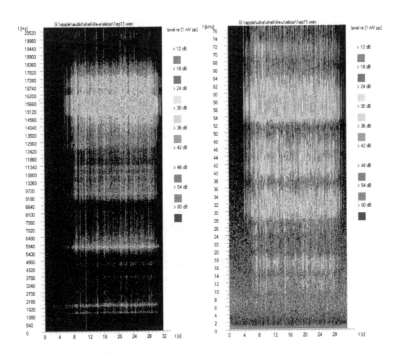

Figure 9. Acustograms of apple tissue in puncture test within frequency range 1-16 kHz (left) and 20-75 kHz (right), f – frequency, t – time (result obtained by the author)

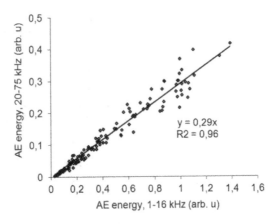

Figure 10. Relationship between the total energy of acoustic signal recorded within frequency range 1-16 kHz and 20-75kHz for apples in puncture test (result obtained by the author)

Fig. 11 presents changes of total AE events and mean AE amplitude during shelf life storage of three apple cultivars. Data was obtained in puncture test. AE descriptors decrease almost linearly during shelf-life storage revealing large Pearson's correlation coefficients R with time of storage (Table 1). In Fig. 11 is visible that the acoustic emission method is very sensitive for registering changes that occur during postharvest storage of apples. Total number of AE events and mean AE amplitude usually shows higher R value when compared to firmness from puncture test (Table 1).

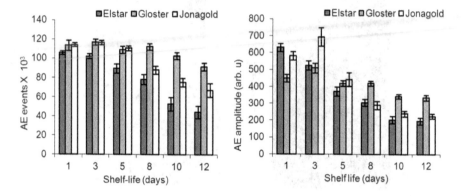

Figure 11. Total number of AE events and mean AE amplitude registered in puncture test of apples (three cultivars) during shelf life storage (result obtained by the author)

Variable	R		
	Elstar	Gloster	Jonagold
AE events	-0,80	-0,54	-0,81
AE amplitude	-0,90	-0,70	-0,88
Firmness	-0,80	-0,40	-0,82

Table 1. Correlation coefficients R of changes of AE events, AE mean amplitude and firmness, in puncture test of apples with shelf-life days for three cultivars 'Elstar', 'Gloster' and 'Jonagold' (results obtained by the author)

The postharvest softening of apples is caused by biochemical processes. During apple ripening two major processes occur that affect the mechanical properties of the tissue including its fracturing mechanism. Pectin degradation during ripening causes a decrease of adhesion between cells leading to tissue softening and changes the fracturing mode toward cell–cell debonding. As a result of respiration and metabolism during storage, turgor pressure can decrease, which has consequences for the fracturing process. The lower tension of the cell wall at low turgor causes a greater deformation that leads to wall fracture. Another consequence of low turgor is a decrease of cell–cell adhesion. Thus, in general, degradation of pectins and lower turgor lead to changes of fracturing mode toward cell–cell debonding. Due to the microstructure, the thin cell wall in plants is considered as an elasto-plastic material. The elasto-plastic character of the cell wall is responsible for the brittle fracturing necessary for sound generation. The intercellular lamella between cells consists of amorphous pectin and are considered as plastic. It is probable that the pectin plasticity causes slow dissipation of strain energy and no brittle fracturing without sound generation. Therefore, it is most likely that the sound made during puncturing is generated mostly when cell walls fracture. In material science terms, a crack propagates if there is a stress concentration into a small tip zone. Thus, propagation is ineffective if there is any plastic zone (in the case of apples it would be pectin). Other features that halt crack propagation are the cell interiors or intercellular spaces. There is ~ 25 % space within apple tissue, and this amount increases with ripening. Thus, ripening attenuates conditions of cracking propagation. Again, in terms of material science, the cell wall (as the material where the stress can concentrate) has a key role in crack propagation.

The maximum number of acoustic events recorded after pushing the probe into the apple flesh was about 10^5 (Fig. 11), which was obtained for fresh apples immediately after harvest. This number agrees roughly with the number of fractured cell walls during the test estimated on the basis of two assumptions; that the mean cell diameter is ~0.25 mm, which is true for apples, and all cells in the path of the probe are damaged (i.e., all cell walls are broken). This result shows that the breakage of each cell wall would be the source of single acoustic event. The mean AE amplitude depends on a stress value in the source of cracking (i.e. the strength of the cell wall) and on the attenuation of the elastic waves on the way from the source to the sensor. As mentioned above, pectin degradation occurs during apple storage, which can decrease the strength of the cell walls due to an increased mobility of cellulose fibrils in the pectin matrix. On the other hand, softening of the bulk tissue caused by pectin degradation in general and the decrease of turgor, increases the attenuation of the elastic waves. Both causes that amplitude decrease with softening of apples.

4.2. Texture Profile Analysis (TPA)

Texture profile analysis (TPA) is used for simulation of eating process. Compression test is performed in two cycles to the same deformation level of a sample. Scheme of TPA test and graphical representation of TPA descriptors used for sample characterization are shown in Fig. 12. Texture profile analysis is performed on cylindrical samples in two cycles. Maximum deformation applied could be about 20-40% of initial sample height for both cycles, depending on sample strength (20% for apple, 40% for potato). Maximum deformation 1 should be close to failure points of investigated material. TPA requires cracking of the test material to simulate the destructive process during eating. On the other hand, deformation should not be too far to prevent the compression of the small pieces of the initial sample in the second cycle which causes springiness and cohesiveness to become physically meaningless. The probe always returns to the trigger point after the first cycle. No rest periods is programmed between the TPA compression cycles to avoid material relaxation. The textural parameters are calculated in the following way (Fig. 12). Hardness 1 is the force peak of the first cycle. Hardness 2 is the force peak of the second cycle. Cohesiveness is calculated as the ratio of the area under the curve of the second cycle to the area under the curve of the first cycle. Springiness is the ratio L2/L1, where L2 is the time or distance from the beginning of the second cycle to hardness 2 point and L1 is the time or distance from the beginning of the test to the hardness 1 point. Acoustic emission during the TPA could be recorded using the same head as for the puncture test described above.

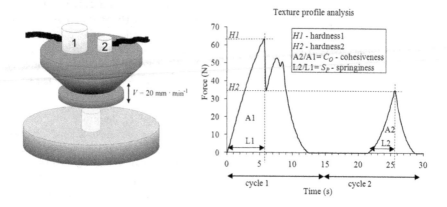

Figure 12. Scheme of TPA test performed on cylindrical sample of plant tissue. Proposed positioning of the AE sensors (1 and 2 with different frequency range) is shown. The upper plate for compression is removable to change a probe for other mechanical tests. Graph to the right presents typical TPA curve with the method of calculation texture descriptors (by the author)

Typical TPA curves together with acoustic emission counts for apple and potato are shown in Fig.13. For comparison, results for two apples, fresh and soft one are plotted, and for hydrated potato sample. The fresh tissue has higher hardness 1 which was reached earlier than in the case of the soft tissue. The range of macro-cracking, visible as the gradual force decrease in the first cycle, is longer and more jagged. The second cycle of TPA also shows larger forces in comparison to soft sample. It is typical that for fresher samples and with higher turgor, the failure occurs at a lower deformation or earlier on the time axis. Acoustic signal appears earlier and it has higher values in the case of fresh apple than in the case of soft one. In apple, acoustic counts are recorded almost from the beginning of the compression. This would be a result of both weaker cell walls and intercellular bonds than for potato which is actually very dense and strong tissue. Failure is accompanied by high acoustic emission counts for both materials as a result of macro-cracking (Fig. 13). This moment is also usually air-conducted and audible. The acoustic emission in TPA is recorded mainly during the downward movement of the machine probe. During the upward movement, a small signal is only observed just after the probe starts returning. It disappears at the end of the returning stage. The second cycle of TPA may also cause acoustic emission. However, the signal is usually weak especially in the case of apple. The second cycle in TPA starts from the trigger point of the first cycle. Thus, the time of deformation during the second cycle is related to recovery of the material after the first cycle. If a crack occurs during the first cycle, it can propagate during the second one. If the material failed during the first cycle (macro-cracking occurred) relaxation of the material is less and deformation in the second cycle is also smaller. Therefore cracking propagation is less and, as consequence, acoustic emission is low. In other words, the weakening of the material in the first cycle causes only small acoustic emission due to the propagation of already existing cracks within the material during the second cycle.

Fig. 14 and Table 2 show decrease of acoustic descriptors during shelf life and that the correlation with days of storage is in general similar as for mechanical descriptors from this test.

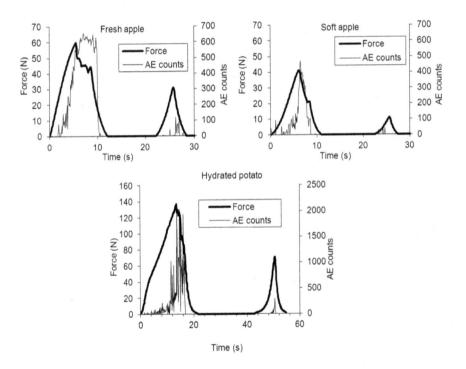

Figure 13. Typical TPA curves with AE counts for fresh and soft apple, and for hydrated potato sample (result obtained by the author)

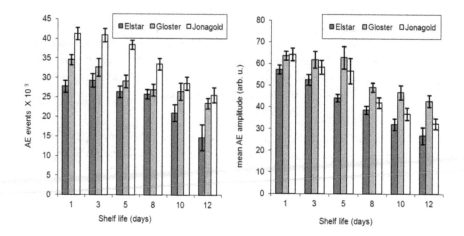

Figure 14. Change of acoustic descriptors obtained in TPA test during shelf life storage for three apple cultivars (result obtained by the author)

Variable	R		
	Elstar	Gloster	Jonagold
AE events	-0,58	-0,64	-0,78
Mean AE amplitude	-0,83	-0,70	-0,82
H1	-0,78	-0,19	-0,85
H2	-0,78	-0,33	-0,83
C_O	-0,45	-0,19	-0,44
S_P	-0,23	0,27	0,38

Table 2. Correlation coefficients between AE events, mean AE amplitude, hardness H1 and H2, cohesiveness C_o, springiness S_P in TPA test and shelf life days for three apple cultivars 'Elstar', Gloster' and 'Jonagold' (result obtained by the author)

4.3. Single edge notched bending (SENB)

Recently, new engineering mechanical tests has been introduced for analysing the fracture properties of plant tissue, so called single edge notched bending (SENB) [9]. In the test rectangular sample with a notch is bended to breaking up. From sample geometry and from failure force obtained from force-bending curve, a critical stress intensity factor K_c can be calculated. This material parameter is tried to correlate with textural properties of a tissue, like crispness or crunchiness. However, from mechanical point of view, the critical stress intensity factor is a force criterion for starting cracking propagation up within material.

Single edge notched bending is performed on rectangular beams according to the ASTM Specification E-399 standard. It is very often that fruit or veggies size or geometry does not allow cutting desired by the standard sample dimensions, which should be also sufficient to produce detectable acoustic emission. According to the standard, S/W=4 (span/height) is suggested [10]. Sample of potato tissue of height W=16 mm and width B=8mm emits strong enough signal in the system showed in Fig. 7 and Fig. 15. Although, to keep the ratio the span should be 64mm, it is usually difficult to cut samples longer than L=40mm from typical potato or apple.. Therefore, the span most often must be shortened to S=32mm for example, which is reasonable and gives S/W=2 ratio. According to standard, in the middle of the sample a notch with depth of a=8mm is cut.

Scheme of SENB test configuration is presented in Fig. 15. Acoustic emission during the SENB could be recorded using the same head as for the puncture test described above where one or more AE sensors could be placed. Sample is placed on support with the notch to the bottom. Bending is performed up to fracture of the sample.

SENB allows determination of a critical stress intensity factor K_c. The K_c can be obtained using formula:

$$K_c = \frac{P_c S}{B W^{\frac{3}{2}}} f\left(\frac{a}{W}\right). \tag{2}$$

where: S- span, P_c is a failure force. Function $f(a/W)$ is given as:

$$f\left(\frac{a}{W}\right) = \frac{3A(\frac{a}{W})^{1/2}}{2\left(1+\frac{2a}{W}\right)(1-\frac{a}{W})^{3/2}}. \tag{3}$$

where:

$$A = 1.99 - a/W(1-\frac{a}{W})(2.15 - \frac{3.93a}{W} + \frac{2.7a^2}{W^2}). \tag{4}$$

K_c has a physical meaning if following formula is true:

$$B_C \geq 2.5(\frac{K_c}{\sigma_y})^2. \tag{5}$$

where: B_c is minimal width of a sample used, σ_y is a failure stress in uniaxial compression of the same material.

Figure 16 presents typical SENB curve and acoustic emission events for fresh and soft apple. AE signal starts just from the beginning of bending which suggest that cracking propagation also starts from the tip of the notch. For fresh apples, which is also harder and has higher K_c value, AE is significantly larger than for the soft material however in both cases acoustic emission lasts up to sample fracture.

SENB test, similar to puncture and TPA, is able to distinguish sample according to its softness. Fig. 17 presents example for three apple cultivars which were stored at shelf life conditions. It is visible that acoustic descriptors diminishes during storage. Table 3 presents correlation coefficients of parameters obtained from SENB test with time of shelf life storage. The coefficients for acoustic descriptors are higher than these for mechanical descriptors which shows again that AE method is very suitable for monitoring properties of fruits.

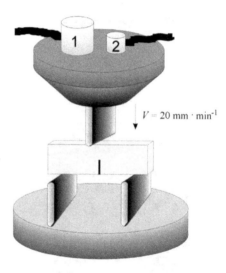

Figure 15. Scheme of the single edge notched bending SENB test for plant tissue with locations of AE sensors (1 and 2, for audible and ultrasound range for example), (by the author)

Variable	R		
	Elstar	**Gloster**	**Jonagold**
AE events	-0,77	-0,43	-0,83
Mean AE amplitude	-0,78	-0,47	-0,84
Work to maximum force	-0,52	-0,14	-0,64
K_c	-0,70	-0,18	-0,73

Table 3. Correlation coefficients R for changes work to maximum force, K_c, AE events, mean AE amplitude in SENB test and days of shelf life for three apple cultivars 'Elstar', 'Gloster' and 'Jonagold' (result obtained by the author)

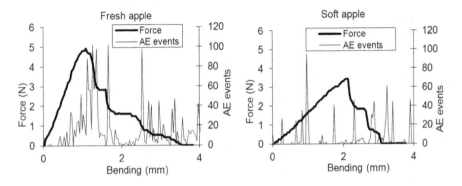

Figure 16. Typical SENB curves with acoustic emission for fresh and soft apples (result obtained by the author)

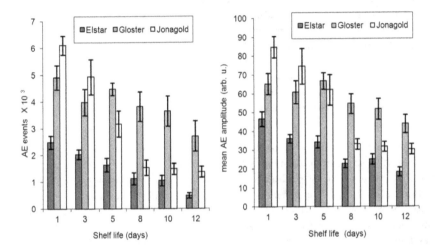

Figure 17. Change of acoustic descriptors obtained in SENB test during shelf life storage for three apple cultivars (result obtained by the author)

5. Evaluation of sensory properties with acoustic emission

There are four key factors of food quality: appearance, smell, texture, and nutritional value [11]. The first three are known as sensory acceptability factors, since they are perceived by the human senses and can be evaluated directly by the consumers. Sensory acceptability of food products is incredibly important, since people want to enjoy eating their favorite products. It can also be difficult to convince consumers to eat healthy products that are unappealing in terms of appearance and texture. Food gives us pleasure not just through its flavour or fragrance; we also want to be aware that what we are eating is fresh. In case of fruit, we associate the latter with mechanical qualities; fruits are desirable when their texture is crunchy, crisp and juicy, and less so when they are mealy.

From a mechanical perspective, crispness, juiciness, and mealiness are all associated with how the cellular structure is broken down. If biting into an apple causes the cell walls to rupture releasing intracellular juices, it makes the apple feel juicy and crispy. This is because of the acoustic signal generated as part of the process, which is perceived positively by our auditory system. It is believed also that crispness can be perceived as a combination of acoustic impressions and the strength required to break down the product, while the acoustic signal is largely perceived as vibrations by the jaw bone (bone-conducted sound). Once the cellular walls rupture, the fruit takes on a mealy quality and the fruit is generally perceived to be overripe.

Texture is a sensory characteristic; assessing it objectively is extremely difficult since consumers' personal and cultural predispositions vary greatly, and perceptions can even depend on the person's mood or frame of mind at the time. Texture of fruits and veggies is also not a constant feature, and is affected by many factors, such as natural biological variability, treatment prior to picking, time of picking, and method and duration of storage. This is why it should be monitored on an ongoing basis, while at the same time the measurements should be simple, repeatable, and low-cost. Unfortunately sensory assessment conducted by a professional panel or representative group of consumers does not meet these criteria.

Since crispness may be the bone-conducted phenomena the approach of utilizing acoustic emission with use of sensor in contact with sample is appropriate way of instrumental analysis of the sensory texture sound-related properties. An advantage of this approach is relatively low sensitivity to external noises comparing to air conducted methods, like these ones which use microphones placed close to sample. The use of the "contact" acoustic emission while mechanical test has also advantage of recording both important for consumers attributes: acoustic and mechanical ones. Typically, system used must be calibrated with reference to standard sensory analysis. Descriptors from instrumental method, independently or as a combination, should be compared with sensory texture attributes to provide the most robust calibration model as possible.

Despite of various mechanical methods used for quality testing of fruits, described previously, the puncture method is still the most popular. This simple puncture test has been used for a long time in laboratories, orchards and industry. The output of the test is firmness value expressed in Newton (N) defined as the maximum force needed to push probe into fruit flesh. In the most common configuration of the test, probe of 11.1 mm with dome-shaped ending with a radius of curvature of 8.73 mm is pushed 8 mm into the fruit. These settings are valid especially for apples. For other fruit they can be adjusted according to their hardness and dimension.

For acoustic emission, the system presented in Fig. 7 may be used. It could be a laboratory system with commercial universal testing machine (machine noise at desired speed should be considered) completed with a low noise set up for AE recording and the most important: correctly chosen sensor. Since the goal is to relate sensory perception with the instrumental method, the frequency range of sensor used can be limited to the audible range: 1-16 kHz. This range can be covered easily by one sensor only. The use of commercial devices provides possibility of easy adjusting of settings to different materials and application of different mechanical loadings programmes, however it is relatively expensive solution. Recently the first simplified system has been developed for apples only (Fig. 18). The CAED (contact acoustic emission detector developed by the author) has a fixed puncture probe and the parameter of the puncture test adjusted exactly for apple. The device uses an accelerometer with sensitivity within the audible frequency range. To avoid large data sets, electronic converts time-amplitude signal into counts in 0.1s time intervals. Counts and actual force can be exported to ASCII whereas sum of all counts (called total AE counts) in the test and firmness are displayed after each test.

A different instrument for texture evaluation was proposed by N. Sakurai's team from Japan (Fig. 19). The device uses a piezoelectric element, attached between wedge type probe for inserting into investigated material and piston driven by hydraulic mechanism [12]. Vibrations, caused by destruction by the wedge type probe of investigated fruit or veggies, are detected by piezoelement. The absolute amplitude in Volts (V) and time of duration of the signal (T) has been used for definition so called Texture Index (TI) according to the formula:

$$TI = \frac{\sum |V|}{T}. \tag{6}$$

TI could be determined within several frequency bands to check witch of them could discriminate a sample. TI has been used for many fruits and vegetables as well for dray food products which showed that TI has frequency related pattern characteristic for different objects. TI was also compared with sensory texture of persimmon which showed that correlation of TI with several texture attributes (sweetness, juiciness, thickness, hardness, fragrance, appearance, and overall acceptability) can reach 0.8, particularly in the frequency range lower than 3 kHz [13].

To calibrate the instrumental method with the use of acoustic emission, a generic descriptive analysis is a suitable method for obtaining sensory texture attributes. Sensory testing laboratory should fulfils the general requirements of a standard, as an example ISO 8589:1988 standard for sensory testing conditions. Each test booth should be equipped with a system for data acquisition from panellists. The expert panel usually consists more than 6 trained persons selected on the basis of the ability of individuals to discriminate tastes and texture attributes. Before the experiment, the panellists usually take part in a training session, where definitions of attributes are discussed and clarified (as in Table 4). For the experiment pieces of fruits are assigned a code and the samples are presented to panellists in random order.

During the experiment the panellists determine the perceived intensity of texture attributes using linear, unstructured scale with a range of 0 – 100 points. After the test, the results are often converted to the most frequently used: 10-point scale.

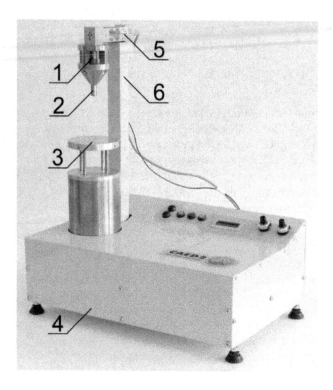

Figure 18. Contact acoustic emission detector (CAED) for apple testing developed by the author. Device uses AE sensor (1) which is placed in the AE head ended by the puncture probe (2). Apple is lift up by a motorized stage (3) to puncture probe. Force is recorded by the force sensor (5) with capacity of 200 N. Electronic (4) calculates on line AE counts and records the actual force within 0.1s time intervals. Sum of counts and firmness (N) are displayed on the screen after the test (photo by the author)

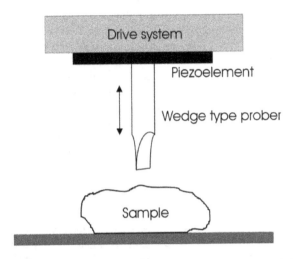

Figure 19. Scheme of device for texture index (TI) evaluation (scheme based on Taniwaki et al. [13])

Sensory texture attribute	Definition	Scale
Crispness	The sound intensity during the first bite with the front teeth	0 = no sound, 100 = very noisy
Hardness	The resistance during the first bite with the front teeth	0 = very soft, 100 = very hard
Juiciness	The sense of juice release during biting	0 = no juice, dry, 100 = very juicy
Mealiness	The mealy sense, especially on the tongue and the palate	0 = not mealy, 100 = very mealy
Overall texture	The overall sensory harmonization of textural attributes	0 = bad, 100 = very good

Table 4. Definitions and scale of some sensory texture attributes.

In the case of CAED which provides mechanical and acoustic indexes, for construction calibration models, several methods can be used: simple linear regression, multiple linear regression or multivariative regressions. For construction the models, averaged values from 10 apples (totally 244 samples from 19 apple cultivars) were taken, as it is usually assumed for sensory analysis to minimalize individual preferences. Examples of statistics for different calibration models are presented in Table 5 (after Zdunek et al. [14]). These data were obtained for different 19 apple cultivars, which were stored in various ways. This example shows that the performances of the linear regression models are satisfactory for crispness and hardness prediction by both firmness or by total AE counts however quantitative prediction is impossible in any case using this modelling approach. Crispness is slightly better predicted by total AE counts than by firmness when these individuals are taken for simple linear model whereas hardness is apparently better predicted by firmness than by acoustic variable. It is presumably due to different origins of the variables: sensory crispness is governed mostly from auditory phenomena whereas sensory hardness from mechanical one. Table 5 presents also performance statistics of multiple regression models (MLR) where both firmness F and total AE counts were considered in the linear model. General improvement of models is observed in the case of each sensory attribute. Furthermore, multivariative principal components regression (PCR) models, where total AE counts and firmness are used as the predictors of a group of sensory variables, show remarkable improvement of calibration performance comparing to linear regression and multiple regression models. Full cross validation (CV) in the PCR for showed that satisfactory prediction is possible in the case of hardness. The models allow for prediction also crispness and overall texture with slightly less accuracy. In the case of juiciness, successful prediction seems to be doubtful whereas mealiness prediction is impossible. Test set validation (TSV) method showed apparently better model performance in the case of crispness and slightly better in the case of juiciness whereas for the rest of sensory attributes performance from TSV method is worse that from CV method. In general both validation methods show satisfactory prediction of crispness and hardness from multivariative PCR calibration models.

The model improvement, when both acoustic and firmness are considered in calibration models, agrees with the hypothesis that crispness perception should be interpreted as counteraction of acoustic and mechanical phenomena. It is usually observed that firmer apples are also more crispy. In Fig. 8 it is visible that firmer apple has more jagged force-deformation (FD) profile during puncturing whereas soft apple has more smoother one. It was accompanied with higher AE counts at the each force dropping down. One can say that firm apple is also more brittle. The jaggedness of the FD is important from the point of view crispness because humans can detect loads of less than 0.1 N. Such interpretation is especially true for dry food stuff however there is no reason to refuse it for plant tissue where sound is produced mainly from cell wall breakdowns and it could cause the momentary force dripping down. It has been shown for dry food that acoustic and mechanical parameters related with saw like force profile could be used for sensory crispness measurement [15], thus presumably in a future it will be the case also for fruits and vegetables.

The above calibration models for CAED were obtained with use of averaged values from 10 apples for the each calibration point. Taking into account that RMSEP value of the calibration models is slightly less than 1, an error of prediction is not larger than ±1. Since descriptive sensory analysis uses the 10 grade scale, the PCR calibration models allow for classification of sensory attribute to one of the 5 grades. This is very satisfactory results taking into account that the results obtained is less expensive and testing of the 10 apples lasts less than 10 minutes only. This means that instrumental evaluation of fruit texture with use of combination of sound-related descriptors and mechanical descriptors could replace soon sensory panels as it is faster, and – as is usually the case with technology – it is objective and does not suffer from fatigue.

Variables used for calibration	Validation method	Performance statistic of validation	Calibrated sensory texture attribute				
			crispness	hardness	juiciness	mealiness	overall texture
Linear regression F	CV	R^2	0.57	0.68	0.40	0.38	0.52
		RMSECV	1.10	0.86	0.95	0.83	1.05
		RPD	1.53	1.75	1.29	1.27	1.45
Linear regression C_{AE}	CV	R^2	0.62	0.60	0.48	0.33	0.52
		RMSECV	0.98	0.95	0.89	0.87	1.06
		RPD	1.72	1.63	1.45	1.27	1.50
Multi-linear regression F and C_{AE}	CV	R^2	0.71	0.77	0.53	0.43	0.62
		RMSECV	0.90	0.73	0.84	0.80	0.96
		RPD	1.87	2.07	1.46	1.32	1.59
Principal component regression F and C_{AE}	CV Ncal=244	R^2	0.72	0.77	0.53	0.43	0.63
		RMSECV	0.90	0.73	0.84	0.80	0.93
		RPD	1.87	2.12	1.53	1.38	1.71
Principal component regression F and C_{AE}	TSV Ncal=187 Ntest=57	R^2	0.90	0.77	0.67	0.25	0.51
		RMSEP	0.53	0.66	0.68	0.96	1.01
		RPD	2.91	2.04	1.61	1.15	1.44

Table 5. Performance statistics of linear regression models, multiple regression and principal component regression models for prediction sensory texture attributes of apples by CAED (after Zdunek et al [14]). Ncal – Number of samples used for calibration. Ntest – Number of samples used for validation, F-firmness, C_{AE} – total AE counts, CV-cross validation, R^2 – determination coefficient, RMSECV - root mean squared errors of cross validation or RMSEP - root mean squared error of prediction, RPD - ratio of prediction to deviation calculated as the ratio of standard deviation of validation data set to RMSECV or RMSEP. If the RPD was below 1.5 the model is not useful, and when the value was higher than 2, the model can predict quantitatively sensory attributes [16]

Author details

Artur Zdunek

Address all correspondence to: a.zdunek@ipan.lublin.pl

Institute of Agrophysics, Polish Academy of Sciences, Lublin, Poland

References

[1] Drake BK. Food Crushing Sounds: An Introductory Study, Journal of Food Science 1963; 28, 233-241.

[2] Chen J, Karlsson C, Povey M. Acoustic envelope detector for crispness assessment of biscuits. Journal of Texture Studies 2005; 36, 139-156.

[3] Vickers Z. Crackliness: Relationships of Auditory Judgments to Tactile Judgments and Instrumental Acoustical Measurements. Journal of Texture Studies; 1983, 15, 49–58.

[4] Christensen CM, Vickers ZM. Relationships of Chewing Sounds to Judgments of Food Crispness. Journal of Food Science 1981; 46, 574.

[5] Fillion L, Kilcast D. Consumer Perception of Crispness and Crunchiness an Fruits and Vegetables. Food Quality and Preference 2002; 13, 23–29.

[6] Zdunek A, Konstankiewicz K. Acoustic emission as a method for the detection of fractures in the plant tissue caused by the external forces International Agrophysics 1997; 11 (3) , 223-227.

[7] Malecki I, Ranachowski J. Acoustic emission, sources, methods, applications. Biuro Pascal, Warsaw; 1984. (in Polish).

[8] Zdunek A, Konstankiewicz K. Acoustic Emission in Investigation of Plant Tissue Micro-Cracking. Transaction of the. ASAE 2004; 47(4), 1171-1177.

[9] Alvarez MD, Saunders DEJ, Vincent JFV, Jeronimidis G. An engineering method to evaluate the crisp texture of fruit and vegetables. Journal of Texture Studies 2000; 31, 457-473.

[10] Williams JG, Cawood MJ. European Group on Fracture: K_c and G_c Methods for Polymer. Polymer Testing 1999; 9, 15-26.

[11] Bourne MC. Food Texture and Viscosity: Concept and Measurement. Second Edition. Academic Press, London; 2002.

[12] Taniwaki M, Hanada T, Sakurai N. Device for Acoustic Measurement of Food Texture Using a Piezoelectric Sensor. Food Research International 2006; 39, 1099–1105.

[13] Taniwaki M, Hanada T, Sakurai N. Postharvest Quality Evaluation of "Fuyu" and "Taishuu" Persimmons Using a Nondestructive Vibrational Method and an Acoustic Vibration Technique, Postharvest Biology and Technology 2009; 51 80–85.

[14] Zdunek A, Cybulska J, Konopacka D, Rutkowski K. Evaluation of Apple Texture with Contact Acoustic Emission Detector: a Study on Performance of Calibration Models. Journal of Food Engineering 2011; 106, 80-87.

[15] Luyten H, Plijter JJ, Van Vliet T. Crispy/Crunchy Crusts of Cellular Solid Foods: a Literature Review with Discussion. Journal of Texture Studies 2004; 35, 445–492.

[16] Saeys W, Mouazen AM, Ramon H. Potential for Onsite and Online Analysis of Pig Manure Using Visible and Near Infrared Reflectance Spectroscopy. Biosystems Engineering 2005; 91 (4), 393–402.

Chapter 9

Otoacoustic Emissions

Giovanna Zimatore, Domenico Stanzial and
Maria Patrizia Orlando

Additional information is available at the end of the chapter

1. Introduction

In this chapter, we present a very special kind of acoustic emissions, coming from inside the cochlea and generated along the basilar membrane by the electro-motile (active) vibrations of outer hair cells of the organ of Corti. They are called OtoAcoustic Emissions (OAE) and are detected in the ear canal by means of microphones which are usually assembled as part of earphone-like probes. Since their discovery by Kemp [1], the study of otoacoustic emissions has become an hot topic both in basic and clinical research, due to OAE unique feature to inform directly about the normal and pathological functions of the cochlear receptors mechanisms, thus like the efficiency of the middle ear transmission chain.

From the signal point of view, the most interesting characteristics of OAE is their broad band frequency spectrum so rousing also a new interest for broad band ear immittance measurements and interpretation [2]. In this respect, this chapter will focus the reader's attention on two very innovative topics to improve objective and non-invasive audiological tests: the potentiality of Transient-Evoked otoacoustic emissions (TEOAE) to detect hearing impairment and the availability of a new microprobe able to capture directly both the pressure and velocity acoustic signals in the ear canal so allowing the direct measurement of ear immittance.

2. Inside cochlea

The cochlea is located in the inner ear, consisting of the front labyrinth and rear labyrinth, the latter having peripheral vestibular formations. The cochlea has quite a complex structure, just as complex as the Organ of Corti, contained inside the cochlea that with its neuro-epithelial hair cells makes up the first mechanical-electrical transformation stage of the sound impulse;

it permits the stimulation of the afferent neural structures and the transmission of the information contained in the sound input through the acoustic canals right up to the cerebral cortex.

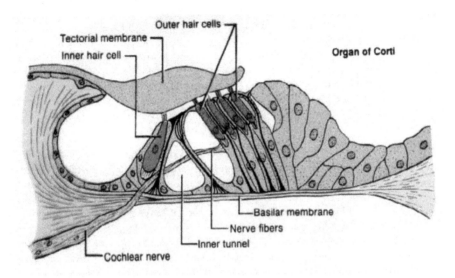

Figure 1. The Organ of Corti The organ of Corti is attached to the basilar membrane on the side of the aqueous fluid of the scala media. It is comprised of the supporting cells for the hair cells, the hair cells themselves, and the tectorial membrane (TM).

The Organ of Corti is made up of the Basilar Membrane, hair cells, support cells, Deiter, Hensen and Claudius cells, and the Tectorial Membrane. The hair cells can be divided according to their position in respect of the cochlea canal, whether outer or inner. The outer cells are more numerous and are placed along three lines; their hairs contact directly with the Tectorial Membrane and are very sensitive, are mainly stimulated by the efferent medial olivocochlea system of control. Acetylcholine (Ach) is their principal chemical mediator. The internal hair cells are arranged in a single line, don't have direct contact with the Tectorial Membrane, are less vulnerable and are supplied by afferent medial olivocochlea nerves, whose first nerve cell is within the Organ of Corti, itself enclosed within the bony labyrinth inside the cochlea. The glutamate is the main neuro–transmitter of the Internal Hair Cells. Given their afferent innervations they make up the actual sensorial cells.

The mechanical-electrical transduction of the cochlea takes place through a series of bio-chemical and bio-mechanical mechanisms. The sound impulse is transmitted from the movement of the stirrup bone on the oval window to the endolymph fluid creating a deformation of the Basilar Membrane on which the Organ of Corti rests with its hair cells that also create a deformation of the auditory cells who in turn are partially in direct contact with the Tectorial Membrane and so generating a deformation wave in the Basilar Membrane (travelling wave) as a result of the sound wave. The amount of deformation that the travelling wave produces along the Basilar Membrane will be evident at different points according to the frequency of the topical tone sound. The result of such mechanical modifications by the Basilar Membrane and hairs is the releasing of neuro-receptor neurohumours located in their synaptic vesicles inside the Hair Cells and so generating the bio-electrical impulse. The Basilar Membrane has different physical and elastic properties along the cochlea spiral from its base, through the intermediate part, to the apex. Even resonance properties vary along the cochlea. This makes one part of the Basilar Membrane resonate and deform according to the frequency of the sound rather than another part of the Basilar Membrane and consequently the Organ of Corti, the activating groups of Hair Cells and their nerve fibres based on the different frequencies contained in the sound. The part of the Basilar Membrane that is most sensitive to low frequency sounds is the apex of the cochlea whilst the part most sensitive to high frequencies is the widest part of the coil that is the base of the cochlea.

The first neuron of the auditory system is contained in the Corti Gland inside the cochlea where we find T cells whose peripheral extensions come from the Internal Hair Cells whilst the central extensions together make up the eighth cranial nerve and connect to the pontini bulb centres. It is important to keep in mind, according to the most recent theories, that inside the Organ of Corti at the External Hair Cell level there is an important active magnifying process of the signal that produces significant amplification, definition and resolution in the frequency of the sound inputs and a notable refinement of the auditory threshold. The fine longitudinal and transversal motility of the Outer Hair Cells, both spontaneous types and those stimulated externally, motility modulated by the efferent olivocochlea system, are the basis of such important functions. From this it can be deduced that a loss of Outer Hair Cells would produce a series of auditory problems more critical and complex in respect of damage to the Inner Hair Cells. Hearing loss (reduction of auditory function) connected to changes in analysis, peripheral translation and conduction of apparatus is defined as neurosensory and gives way to distortions in frequency, intensity such as recruitment, a phenomenon that distorts the subjective sound intensity (loudness), in phase, exertion and auditory conformation.

Outer Hair Cells are cells that belong to and are controlled by the efferent system more than sensor cells. They are more sensitive to auditory stimulation in respect of Internal Hair Cells which are anatomically connected to the afferent or sensorial system as previously stated. The particular sensitivity is mainly mechanical in nature and Is connected to 1) the presence of direct tectorial hair connections between stereohairs and the Tectorial Membrane and 2) their "active" vibratory motility, electrically and chemically mediated, that translates into acoustic phenomenon that can be picked up and recorded by a microphone positioned in the external auditory canal: the Otoacoustic Emissions.

3. What OAE are

The discovery of otoemissions is attributed to the English physics professor David Kemp at the end of the '70s. He is merited with first putting forward the idea and then introducing clinical diagnosis using investigative methodologies capable of non-invasive exploration, in humans, the Organ of Corti functions and in particular the Outer Hair Cells. The basis of this methodology has produced a series of new and surprising evidence regarding the cochlea physiology that integrates, contradicts and supersedes the consolidated theories of von Békésy, Nobel Prize winner in 1960.

The direct contact between the stereo cilias of the Outer Hair Cells and the Tectorial Membrane create mechanical-electrical type reactions that transfer to the entire cell connected by ATP (Adenosin-TriPhosfate). The typical cytoskeleton-like network of muscle (actina–miosina) of which the cell is made, makes use of the electric charge originated at the level of the stereo cilia and moves either slowly or rapidly. These movements are modulated and regulated by the medial olivocochlea system, a true servo-system of control through various synaptic neurohumours and in particular Acetylcholine. The function of Outer Hair Cells is fundamental in conferring on our hearing the elevated threshold characteristics, the increased dynamics between minimum audible threshold and the perceptible maximum and frequency selectiveness.

A cochlea system with dysfunctional Outer Hair Cells rapidly loses these properties even if in theory the Inner Hair Cells are healthy. The information received mechanically from the Outer Hair Cells is transmitted in electric form as well as in mechanical form to the Inner Hair Cells and so to our proper sensory auditory system. To stress again, the Outer Hair Cells are particularly vulnerable, their high characteristic sensitivity to which are connected elevated bioenergetic and metabolic requests such that any cochlea noxae that is infected, toxic, traumatised or suffering from a metabolic disorder can bring about a lesion and become apparent prematurely. The study of Otoacoustic emissions appears significant and effective in the majority of auditory problems of peripheral receptors.

The otoacoustic emissions (OAE) are recorded by a particular probe positioned in the external auditory canal. If it is necessary to create responses the probe, other than being a receiver that records the emissions from the cochlea, contains a transducer capable of sending stimuli to the cochlea. These days it is possible to study the OAE mainly in one of three ways:

1. Recording the spontaneous emissions produced by the cochlea in the absence of any acoustic stimulus. Such emissions are called 'Spontaneous Otoacoustic Emissions' (SOAE).

2. Recording the emissions produced inside the cochlea through the sending of temporary acoustic stimuli, such as clicks, that are able to involve synchronously and globally a large number of the acoustic cells from the base to the apex. These emissions are known as 'Transient Otoacoustic Emissions' (TEOAE).

3. Cochlea emissions created by pairs of tonal stimuli of differing frequency for intermodulation phenomena, so-called 'Distortion Product Otoacoustic Emissions' (DPOAE).

Apart from the SOAE method of recording whose clinical value is unfortunately less, we shall focus on the TEOAE and DPOAE recording methods. The first method involves sending a series of clicks from a probe and recording the acoustic response from the hair cells. The acoustic response is normally represented graphically by oscillations based on a time period (milliseconds), as well as by a spectrogram that traces the size and frequency of the response. The DPOAE instead operates by way of sending a pair of pure tones (F1 and F2), with very small value frequency differences between them for example F1=1000 Hz, F2=1220 Hz, a ratio of F2/F1 = 1.22. The two tones, so-called primary tones, give rise to distortions in the cochlea deriving from their combination. The phenomenon of the combination of tones is mostly connected to the peripheral processing mechanisms of the signal which is still not wholly understood but that resides in the internal ear and in particular is connected to the active processes of the cochlea. So if two tones of differing frequency are sent simultaneously, the ear might perceive one or more tones superimposed that are the sum of the two tones or else are the difference (simple, cubic, quadratic, etc.) of the two primary tones. The response traces the form of a DP-gram, showing the extent of the response derived from the frequency of the primary tones.

Nowadays the major diagnostic clinical function is mostly engaged in the TEOAE and DPOAE being the spontaneous emissions less subject to interpretation despite having a notable scientific interest. Dedicated software systems permit the execution of a rapid measurement statistically adapted to the cochlea response. As regards the DPOAE it is interesting to note that it establishes a modern method to survey one of the more characteristic psychoacoustic phenomena: combination tones. The study of DPOAE in particular allows the design of cochlea responses in an audiometric-like way, frequency by frequency, on a graph that shows on the vertical axis the frequencies of stimulation and on the horizontal axis the intensity levels of the received Otoacoustic emissions showing immediately if the audiological threshold is within normal limits or not.

The operating range is important in identifying the dysfunction of the cochlea in Ménière's disease, in evaluating damage from noise, in ototoxic type changes, in the study of some genetic and immunological cochlea alterations, in the differential cochlea diagnosis against retro cochlea diagnosis and the identification of new pathologies such as Auditory Neuropathy. Finally, the range of neonatal auditory screening establishes the most sensitive and specific means of recognising premature infantile deafness. Auditory screening is carried out at birth before the new-born baby is discharged from hospital normally the second day after birth and, given the simplicity and speed of testing, is the best method for definitive diagnosis or alerting and preparing for further diagnosis and rehabilitative therapy within a few months and before the child's first birthday, a period of great neuroplastic and linguistic activity. It's therefore possible to control and limit the damage from auditory sensorial deprivation, language disorders, communication and behaviour disorders.

OAEs provide objectivity and greater accuracy, representing a non invasive tool for the assessment of OHC and the functionality of the cochlear amplifier, as demonstrated by experimental and clinical studies [3-5]; furthermore, the cochlear effects of exogenous factors, such as ototoxic drugs, solvents and high-level sound exposure [6-8], can be monitored by OAE. It has been suggested that OAEs may provide early indication of cochlear damage before evidence for NIHL appears in pure-tone audiometry [9-10]. Recently, TEOAE have been used to study in tinnitus subjects with normal hearing to assess whether a minor cochlear or efferent dysfunction might play a role in tinnitus [11].

One of the few limitations of OAE is related to the extent of hearing loss that we can explore: infact, already for cochlear hearing loss above 50 dB the OAE, just because otoacoustic emissions are produced by the activation of CCE, are no longer evoked.

4. TEOAE recording

To record the TEOAE signals the Otodynamic Analyzer (ILO92, Otodynamics Ltd, Hatfield, United Kingdom), was widely used, by inserting a SGS-type general purpose TEOAE probe into the external ear canal. The TEOAE recordings were carried out in a standard hospital room, corresponding to the usual clinical setting for these measurements. The automated differential non-linear test paradigm was used: the stimulus was characterized by a train of four clicks, three with the same amplitude and polarity, followed by a fourth one with a 3-fold amplitude and opposite polarity with respect to the preceding ones. The 80 μs clicks presented at 50/s were 75–85 dB SPL. The responses were obtained evaluating an average among 260 stimuli trains (1040 clicks) stored into two different buffers (A and B) for a total of 2080 clicks. The value of the automatically computed correlation or reproducibility between the two obtained waveforms (A and B) of an OAE signal is named Repro or whole waveform reproducibility (REPRO) (Pearson correlation coefficient *100) (see in Figure 2, on the right, Repro=99%).

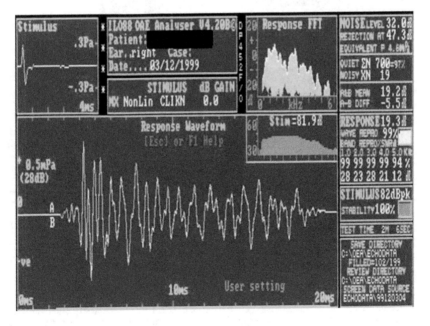

Figure 2. TEOAE signals (ILO92, Otodynamics Ltd)

5. Broad band measurement of ear immittance and perspective for improving TEOAE detection

The most innovative application of micro-electro-mechanical systems (MEMS) technology to acoustic sensors is the manufacturing of thermo-acoustic velocimeters based on the two-wire anemometric transduction principle. These new sensors allow to capture directly the acoustic particle velocity signal v, and thus, by coupling and assembling them with standard micro-phones which are instead sensitive to the pressure signal p, a new generation of pressure-velocity (p-v) micro-probes is nowadays made available (see Figure 3).

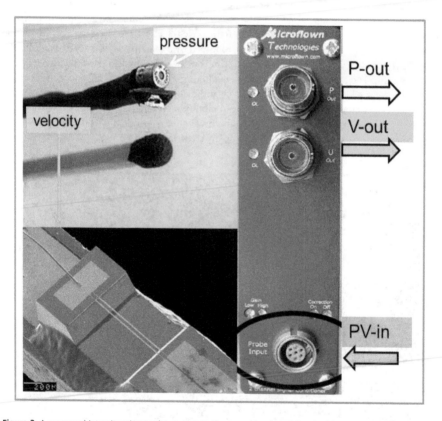

Figure 3. A p-v sound intensity micro-probe consists in the assembly of a miniaturized pressure microphone and a MEMS technology based velocimeter in a single measurement system. While the pressure sensor is a standard electret one, the velocity signal is transduced thanks to the differential anemometric principle applied to two closely spaced heated wires 10 µm apart, 1mm long and 5µm large suspended in parallel in order to form a bridge. The wire composition is 200 nm platinum (Pt) on a silicon nitride (Si3N4) substratum 150 nm thick. The captured pressure and velocity analog signals are conditioned through a common probe input and handled in output as two separate voltage signals. (The commercial system shown in the figure is by courtesy of Microflown®: www.microflown.com).

These micro-probes are clearly the ideal device for carrying out advanced direct measurements of the sound field energetic properties like sound intensity j=pv or acoustic impedance Z=p/v. To this aim, an accurate calibration procedure [12] is needed (see Figure 4).

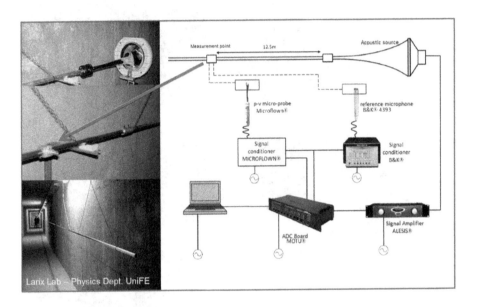

Figure 4. The facility for sound intensity micro-probes calibration installed at the Larix Lab of the Physics Department of University of Ferrara consists in a 48 m long wave guide where a progressive plane wave is generated through a bi-conical loudspeaker in the [50, 10000] Hz frequency range. The p-v micro-probe under calibration is inserted at a distance of 12.5 m from the source and is calibrated by comparison with a reference pressure microphone using the correction function $\Gamma(\omega)$ defined in Equation 13 of Ref. [12].

Of course, the calibration filtering process can be implemented at post-processing level but, with few engineering effort, the calibration filters can also be programmed at hardware level so making, in particular, the measurement of acoustic impedance, a completely automatic task. The technological innovation driven by MEMS application to acoustic sensors can be easily transferred to audiometric devices so transforming for instance a traditional tympanometric probe in a new setup for p-v tympanometry (see Figure 5). The main advantages of a p-v tympanometric test with respect to a traditional one are: a) the direct measure of ear immitance for more precise results; b) the test is completely non-invasive for static pressure external pumping is no longer necessary (p-v test measurements are performed in standard pressure conditions); c) the test produces wideband results in the typical frequency range of multi-tonal tympanometry [100, 1200] Hz; d) the p-v audiometer provides sophisticated sound energy analysis capability for hearing models validation (see Ref. [13]).

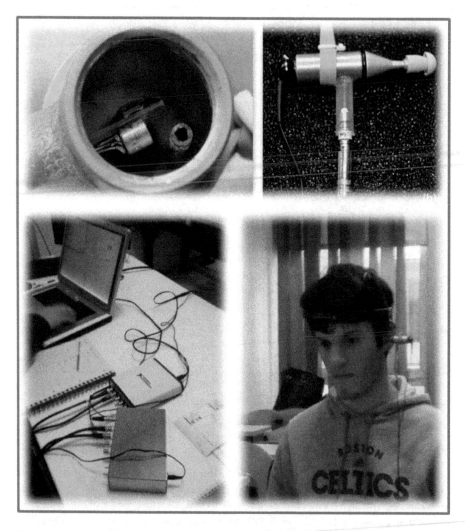

Figure 5. A p-v tympanometer is designed as a laptop based dual channel analyzer (lower left) able to record both the Impulse Responses (IRs) of pressure and velocity signals captured with the p-v tympanometric probe shown in the upper part of the figure. Once the p-v IRs of the ear canal have been measured in atmospheric pressure condition (lower right), the system calculates the external/middle ear specific immittance and displays its magnitude in dB relative to the frequency dependent baseline Y_0 obtained by plugging up the probe.

As an example of results obtained with p-v tympanometry, wideband p-v tympanograms measured in dB for 26 left and right normal ears belonging to 13 voluntary students are clustered and reported in Figure 6.

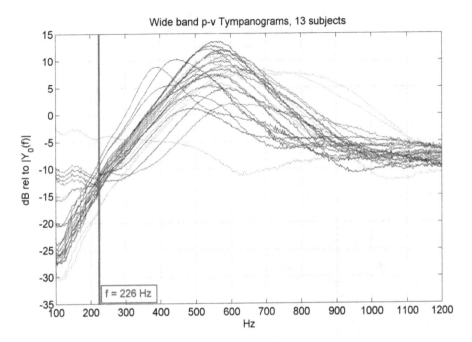

Figure 6. Wideband p-v tympanograms measured in dB for 26 left and right normal ears belonging to 13 voluntary students. One clearly see that all tympanograms converges between -10 and -15 dB for the standard frequency of 226 Hz used in traditional tympanometry. The mean value found at -12.7 dB can thus be considered the "normal" value of the immitance magnitude measured by p-v tympanometry at 226 Hz.

As the primary data collected by the p-v tympanometry are basically the measurement of the pressure and velocity ear canal IRs, a completely new perspective also for OAE studies is also opened. Specifically for the TEOAEs which could be simply detected as the non-linear byproducts of DSP algorithms used in the ear-canal immitance function calculations.

6. TEOAE post-processing analysis

The Recurrence Quantification Analysis (RQA) and Principal Component Analysis (PCA) have been carried on TEOAE waveforms [14-17] (Zimatore et al. 2000, 2001 2002, 2003) to extract new descriptors that could enlighten an early diagnosis of hearing loss.

In the last few years, a new parameter has been introduced to analyse TEOAE, to improve the specificity of diagnostic tests and to reduce inter-subject variability. The work was concentrated on the analysis of the TEOAE focusing on their dynamics by the Recurrence Quantification Analysis (RQA). RQA is a post-processing analysis that is extremely fit to non-stationary signals and represents a valid alternative to Wavelet analysis used by other researchers. In fact, the embedding procedure allows to expand a mono-dimensional signal into multidimensional space, thus permitting the identification of fine peculiarities of the sampled series that in turn are described by few global parameters allowing for a synthetic patient description.

RQA in summary:

- RQA introduces few parameters descriptive of the global complexity of a signal, starting from what is called "recurrence plot"

- RQA descriptors are calculated on the basis of the number and location of dots in the recurrence plot

- RQA dynamic features are independent from signal amplitude

The results obtained demonstrate how proposed new global index can recognize even mild hearing loss and that an assessment of the severity of cochlear damage can be realized.

To build the recurrence plot, the time behavior of the original signal was represented by a series of 512 points equally spaced in time (e.g. {a1 a2 .... a 512} where ai represents the value of the signal corresponding to the i-th time position). Then, the series was arranged in successive columns (the columns number is defined by the "embedding dimension" parameter, N), each-one obtained by applying a delay in time (lag parameter) to the original sequence, in this way an "embedding matrix" was created.

Finally, the recurrence plot was built, drawing a black dot (named "recurrent point") in the represented space if the distance between the corresponding rows (the distance between the j-th and the (j+1)th row is of the embedding matrix was lower than a fixed value (radius). In the obtained plot, the horizontal and vertical axes represented the relative position of the 512 points into the TEOAE waveform. RQA descriptors were then calculated on the basis of the number and the location of dots in the recurrence plot. In particular, percent of recurrence (Rec) is the percentage of recurrence points in a recurrent plot; percent of determinism (Det) is the percentage of recurrence points which form diagonal lines and it indicates the degree of deterministic structure of the signal; entropy (Ent) is the Shannon entropy of the probability distribution of the diagonal line lengths and is linked to the richness of deterministic structure [16-17] (Zimatore et al. 2002 and 2003). The presence of horizontal and vertical lines in the recurrence plot shows that part of the considered signal matches closely with a sequence farther along the time (for more details see http://www.recurrence-plot.tk).

In TEOAE analysis the delay in the embedding procedure (lag) is set to 1; the number of the embedding matrix columns (embedding dimension) is set to 10; and the cut-off distance (radius) is set to 15; to eliminate the initial linear ringing, the first 2.8 ms of the recorded TEOAE signals are excluded.

Comparing Figure 7 and 8, it is clear that recurrence plots distinguish between normal hearing and impaired hearing TEOAEs especially in terms of a reduction in the deterministic structure.

As a further step of the post-processing analysis, the well known Principal Component Analysis (PCA), was applied on the obtained RQA descriptors. Briefly, PCA is a common statistical technique which provides the possibility to reduce the starting data set dimension

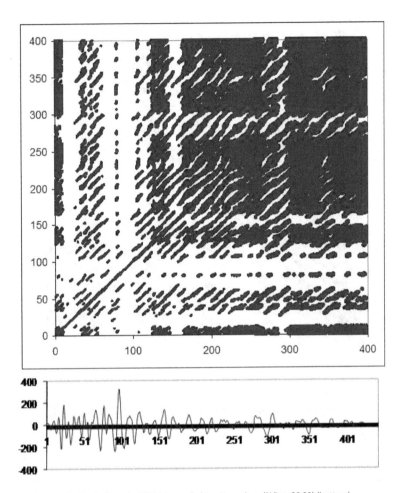

Figure 7. Recurrence plot (top) of a typical TEOAE recorded in a Normal ear (%Det=88.89) (bottom)

without consistent loss of information and with a separation of the different and independent features characterizing the data set. PCA describes the original data set with a lower number of new parameters named main components (PC1, PC2) which explain more than 90% of the total variability in the data set. Having, by construction, PC1 and PC2 zero mean and standard deviation equal to 1, if a set of TEOAE signals from normal ears are studied, 96% of them will fall within a circle centered in the origin of the PC1/PC2 plane, and with a radius equal to 2 (reference circle in figure 12). The PC1/PC2 plane is defined starting from a representative data set made by 118 signals measured from normal hearing subjects [18]. The representative data set was used to define the circle in the PC1/PC2 plane in which the majority of TEOAE signals recorded in normal hearing subjects will fall. Mathematically, the parameter RAD2D is defined

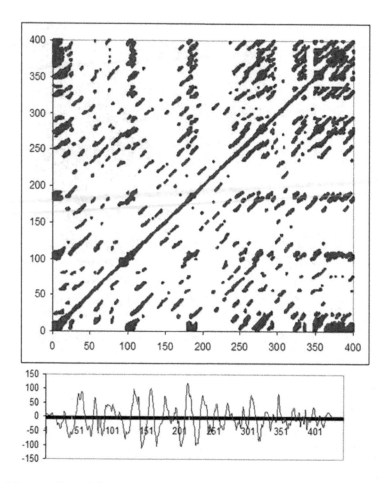

Figure 8. Recurrence Plot (top) of a representative Impaired Hearing (IH) TEOAE waveform (bottom) (% Det = 62.89)

in the PC1/PC2 plane as the Euclidean distance of one point representing a TEOAE signal from the plane origin.

The relation correlating the RAD2D obtained for all the measured signals with the entity of cochlear damage is tested. Specifically, RAD2D was evaluated for real TEOAEs by applying the same procedure as for simulated signals combining RQA and PCA techniques.

Furthermore, the post-processing analysis proposed is useful in screening of adults, in longitudinal studies, in test to evaluate the efficacy of new pharmacological treatments, in conservation program in presbycusis and in protection program in noise induced hearing losses.

Figure 10 illustrates REPRO plotted *vs* RAD2D considering 30 subjects from Florence area (Italy). The examined ears will be classified as normal hearing (NORM) or mild hearing losses

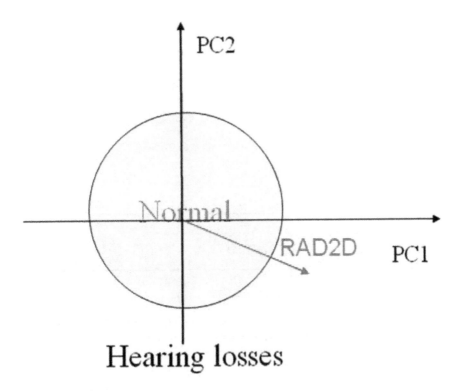

Figure 9. RAD2D is defined in the Principal Components plane as the Euclidean distance from the plane origin; the points representing the normal TEOAE signals fall in the yellow reference circle and TEOAE signals recorded form subjects with hearing losses fall outside.

(MHL) or (severe) hearing losses (HL) ears according to their pure tone thresholds at 0.250, 0.500, 1, 2, 3, 4, 6 and 8 kHz. The three groups according to the maximum hearing threshold level are: NORM, with threshold <10 dB at all audiometric frequencies, MHL, with threshold <20 dB at all audiometric frequencies and >10 dB at least at one frequency, and HL, with threshold >20 dB at least at one frequency. In Figure 10 the HL patients (white circles), in the MHL patients (blue diamonds) and in NORM subjects (black diamonds): each point corresponds to the recorded TEOAE waveform. A very simple and immediate description is available by observing the areas identified by threshold of REPRO (the horizontal line at 70%) and of RAD2D (the vertical line at 1.78). The points above the horizontal line indicate pass signals. To the left side of the vertical line, the points indicate signals that fall inside the normality circle, that is pass signals;. the main result is illustrated in the right upward rectangle of Figure 9 where the ears that have both high REPRO and high RAD2D are shown: these points-signals indicate 8 ears (3 HL, 4 MHL and 1 NORM) screened as pass by REPRO but identified as "fail" by our TEOAE parameter (possible false-negative of ILO test).

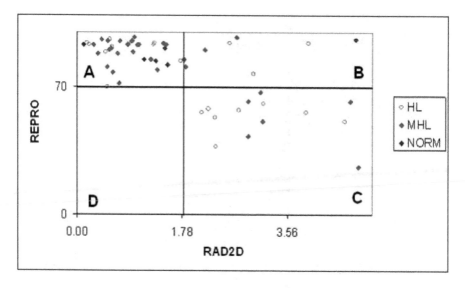

Figure 10. REPRO vs RAD2D from RQA parameters of TEOAE signals

The 8 points-signals that fall in the B area correspond to 8 different subjects: 6 are hunters or they shoot for hobby and 2 work often with tractors or lawn mowers. The combined use of the two global parameters REPRO and RAD2D can enlighten points corresponding to the subjects with high risk of environmental noise exposure.

In this chapter the application of technique such as RQA is proposed because, it allows the quantification of the *fine-structure* of TEOAE signals without any *a priori* hypothesis and any data manipulation; moreover, the dynamical structure of signals can be investigated without taking into account the signal-amplitude differences.

7. TEAOA simulation by mechanistic model

An electronic model of human hearing system is used to test and improve new hypothesis of cochlear mechanisms and to anatomically distinguish different contributions to ear pathologies [18-19].

An electronic model of human hearing system can be used to test and improve new hypothesis of cochlear mechanisms and to anatomically distinguish different contributions to ear pathologies.

The considered ear model is directly inspired to the so called "travelling wave" representation of the cochlear function mechanism and is able to simulate the TEOAE responses; the electric model of the whole ear, originally introduced by Guiguère and Woodland [20-21] and used in

TEOAEs analysis [15, 18, 22], has been implemented into PSpice®. PSpice® is a standard electrical simulation tool for dc, transient and ac analyses [23] (see Figure 11). The input circuit can be defined by using a graphical interface or by compiling a list representing the circuit topology. The outputs of the system are current and voltage values within the circuit which can be displayed in both tabular and graphical formats. PSpice® has been already used to study an electric model of the cochlea [24] due to the possibility to relate the model parameters to physical and physiological issues. In [24], the used lumped parameter model is entirely passive, made of a resistive network combined with two capacitances in order to model the Reissner's membrane and the OHC in the Corti Organ.

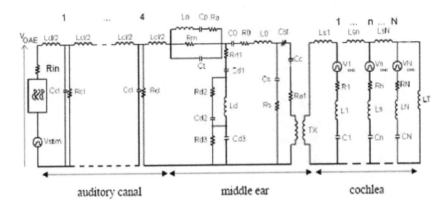

Figure 11. The electronic ear model

The considered ear model is depicted in figure 11 and encompasses the human ear anatomy from the auditory canal to the OHC within the cochlea. The auditory canal is represented by a cascade of four T-sections, corresponding to the segmented form of a uniform transmission line, while the middle ear is modeled as a complex electrical network based on its functional anatomy [25]. An ideal transformer connects the middle ear to the cochlea, to represent the acoustic transformer ratio between the eardrum and the oval window [20-21]. Finally, the cochlea is modeled as a non-uniform and non-linear transmission line, divided into several sections from the base to the apex, each one consisting of a series inductor, a shunt resonant circuit (composed of a resistor, an inductor, and a capacitor), and a non-linear voltage source. In the electro-acoustic analogy, the series inductors represent the acoustic mass of the cochlear fluids; the resistors, inductors and capacitors forming the shunt resonant circuits represent the acoustic resistance, mass and stiffness of the basilar membrane, respectively, and the non linear voltage sources represent the OHC active processes. Finally, the helicotrema is modeled by the inductor LT. The initial values of the electric ear model components are those reported in Table 1 of [20] and also used in [22]. Correspondingly, the cochlea was represented by 128 and 64 partitions [19]

To verify the hypothesis that TEOAE are strongly modulated by the middle ear [17], some elements in the middle ear section were varied according to the experimental study of Avan and colleagues [4]. The first change is the addition of a stapes capacitor (C_{st}) to the middle-ear section of the circuit, as already considered by [20] Giguère and Woodland (1994a) and by [25]. When C_{st} has a large value, its impedance is small, corresponding to small tension in the stapedius muscle (C_{st} equal to infinity corresponds to no stiffness in the resting condition). Conversely, when C_{st} is small, its impedance is large, corresponding to high muscle tension. Then, changes in the tympanic membrane stiffness (C_0, C_{d1}), to account for changes in the middle ear pressure, and in the tympanic membrane mass (L_0, L_d), to simulate an additive mass, have been considered [4]. Furthermore, a dead cochlea condition has been simulated by de-activating the voltage sources in all cochlear sections.

The role of middle ear effects is a hot topic in the OAE field, and would be of high interest to audiology and hearing researchers.

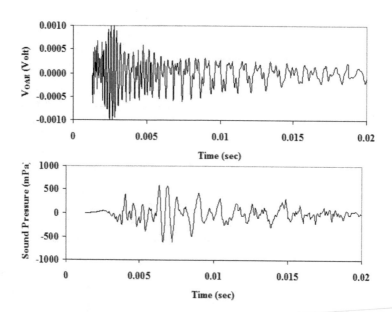

Figure 12. TEOAE Simulated (top) and real (bottom) in normal ear

Figure 12 (top) reports a typical simulated signal, and a real TEOAE signal recorded from a normoacousic subject is reported in figure 12 (bottom). In both simulated and real signals, recording starts after 2.5 ms from the initial external excitation (t = 0), to get rid of the initial ringing. Both signals show oscillations lasting up to 20 ms, with higher frequencies having shorter latency than lower frequencies, in agreement with the latency-frequency relationship typical of TEOAEs. In fact, according to the place–frequency (tonotopic) effect characteristic of the basilar membrane, each element of the membrane acts as a resonator at a frequency inversely proportional to its distance from the oval window.

A very important goal in prevention and clinical applications is to improve the specificity of diagnostic tests and to reduce inter-subject variability in TEOAE signals. A new pass/fail test could be useful for screening but the quantification of cochlear damage is of great interest in research programs. To determine the amount of damage, an ear model can be used to simulate different levels of cochlear damage by silencing a growing number of cochlear partitions. The relation between a new parameter and the number of silenced partitions in the model was evaluated.

From the comparison between the real and simulated RAD2D values it is possible to extrapolate the corresponding number of "hypothetical silenced partitions". In this way, since each partition corresponded to a specific portion of uncoiled cochlea and to a specific number of outer hair cells, a descriptor of OHC integrity is obtained [26].

8. Conclusion

A very important goal in prevention and clinical applications is to improve the specificity of diagnostic tests and to reduce inter-subject variability in TEOAE signals. The availability of new micro-probes able to pick up both the pressure and the air particle velocity signals inside the ear canal, while allowing to update the standard multi-tonal tympanometry with the wideband implementation of p-v tympanometric non-invasive tests, points also to record and analyze TEOAEs as the non-linear by-product of DSP algorithms used in the ear-immitance function computing process. Furthermore, to prevent and to mitigate noise and aging effects on cochlea, a new post-processing procedure could be employed in *longitudinal studies* [27] as well as to test the efficacy of new pharmacological treatments and the opportunity to follow a subject over time.

Author details

Giovanna Zimatore[1], Domenico Stanzial[2] and Maria Patrizia Orlando[1]

*Address all correspondence to: domenico.stanzial@cnr.it

1 CNR-IDASC – Institute of Acoustics and Sensor "Orso Mario Corbino", Rome, Italy

2 CNR-IDASC - Institute of Acoustics and Sensor "Orso Mario Corbino", c/o Physics Department University of Ferrara, Italy

References

[1] Kemp DT. Stimulated acoustic emissions from within the human auditory system," J Acous. Soc Am. 1978;64 1386-1391.

[2] Keefe DH, Folson RC, Gorga MP, Vohr BR, Bulen JC, Norton et al. Identification of Neonatal Hearing Impairment: Ear-Canal Measurements of Acoustic Admittance and Reflectance in Neonates. Ear & Hearing 2000;21(5) 443-461.

[3] Probst R, Lonsbury-Martin BL, Martin GK.. A review of otoacoustic emissions. Journal of the Acoustical Society of America 1991;89 2027-2067.

[4] Avan P, Buki B, Maat B, Dordain M, and Wit HP. Middle ear influence on otoacoustic emissions. I: Non invasive investigation of the human transmission apparatus and comparison with model results Hearing Research 2000;140 189-201.

[5] Avan P and Bonfils P.. Distortion-product otoacoustic emission spectra and high-resolution audiometry in noise-induced hearing loss. Hearing Research 2005;209 (1-2) 68-75.

[6] Uchida Y Ando F , Shimokat, H et al. The Effects of Aging on Distortion-Product Otoacoustic Emissions in Adults with Normal Hearing. Ear & Hearing 2008;29(2) 176-184.

[7] Hamdan AL, Abouchacra KS, Al Hazzouri AGZ.Transient-evoked otoacoustic emissions in a group of professional singers who have normal pure-tone hearing thresholds. Ear and Hearing 2008;29(3) 360-377.

[8] Cianfrone G, Pentangelo D, Cianfrone F, Mazzei F, Turchetta R, Orlando MP, Altissimi G. Pharmacological Drugs Inducing ototoxicity, vestibular symtoms and tinnitus: a reasoned and updated guide. European Review for Medical and Pharmacological Sciences 2011;15 601-636.

[9] Attias J, Furst M, Furman V et al. Noise-induced otoacoustic emission loss with or without hearing loss. Ear Hear 1995;16 612-8.

[10] Shupak A, Tal D, Sharoni Z, et al. Otoacoustic Emissions in Early Noise-Induced Hearing Loss. Otology & Neurotology 2007;28 745-752.

[11] Paglialonga A, Fiocchi S, Del Bo L, Ravazzani P and Tognola G.Quantitative analysis of cochlear active mechanisms in tinnitus subjects with normal hearing sensitivity: time–frequency analysis of transient evoked otoacoustic emissions and contralateral suppression. Auris Nasus Larynx 2011;38(1) 33-40.

[12] Stanzial, 2011 Stanzial D., Sacchi G., Schiffrer G., Calibration of pressure-velocity probes using a progressive plane wave reference field and comparison with nominal calibration filters, J. Acoust. Soc. Am 2011;129 (6) 3745-3755.

[13] Stanzial 2012 Stanzial D, Sacchi G, Schiffrer G. On the physical meaning of the power factor in acoustics, J. Acoust. Soc. Am 2012;131(1) 269-280.

[14] Zimatore G, Giuliani A, Parlapiano C. et al.. Revealing deterministic structures in click-evoked otoacoustic emissions. Journal of Applied Physiology 2000;88(4) 1431-1437.

[15] Zimatore G. The speaking ear. Analysis and modelling of Otoacoustic emissions. PhD thesis in Biophysics, Sapienza University, Rome, 2001.

[16] Zimatore G, Hatzopoulos S, Giuliani et al. Comparison of transient otoacoustic emission responses from neonatal and adult ears. Journal of Applied Physiology 2002;92(6) 2521-2528.

[17] Zimatore G, Hatzopoulos S, Giuliani et al. Otoacoustic emissions at different click intensities: invariant and subject dependent features. Journal of Applied Physiology 2003;95 2299-2305.

[18] Zimatore G, Cavagnaro M, Giuliani A, Colosimo A. Human acoustic fingerprints. Biophysics & Bioengineering Letters 2008;1(2) 1-8.

[19] Zimatore G, CavagnaroM, Giuliani A, Colosimo A. Reproducing Cochlear Signals by a Minimal Electroacoustic Model. Open Journal of Biophysics, 2012;2: 33-39 http://www.SciRP.org/journal/ojbiphy (accessed 7 April 2012)

[20] Giguère C, and Woodland PC. A computational model of the auditory periphery for speech and hearing research. I. Ascending path J. Acoust. Soc. Am 1994;95(1) 331-342.

[21] Giguère C and Woodland PC. A computational model of the auditory periphery for speech and hearing research. II. Descending paths J. Acoust. Soc. Am 1994;95(1) 343-349.

[22] Zheng L, Zhang YT Yang FS et al. Synthesis and decomposition of transient-evoked otoacoustic emissions based on an active auditory model. IEEE Transaction on Biomedical Engineering 1999;46(9) 1098-1105.

[23] PSPICE 1997 PSPICE A/D User's Guide. Irvine CA: Microsim Corp. Version 8.0

[24] Suesserman MF and Spelman FA. Lumped-Parameter Model for In Vivo Cochlear Stimulation. IEEE Trans on Biomed Eng 1993;40(3) 237-245.

[25] Lutman ME and Martin AM Development of an electroacoustic analogue model of the middle ear and acoustic reflex J. of Sound and Vibration 1979;64(1) 133-157.

[26] Zimatore G, Fetoni AR, Paludetti G, Cavagnaro et al.. Post-processing analysis of transient-evoked otoacoustic emissions to detect 4 kHz-notch hearing impairment – a pilot study. Med Sci Monit 2011;17(6) MT41-49.

Permissions

The contributors of this book come from diverse backgrounds, making this book a truly international effort. This book will bring forth new frontiers with its revolutionizing research information and detailed analysis of the nascent developments around the world.

We would like to thank Wojciech Sikorski, PhD, for lending his expertise to make the book truly unique. He has played a crucial role in the development of this book. Without his invaluable contribution this book wouldn't have been possible. He has made vital efforts to compile up to date information on the varied aspects of this subject to make this book a valuable addition to the collection of many professionals and students.

This book was conceptualized with the vision of imparting up-to-date information and advanced data in this field. To ensure the same, a matchless editorial board was set up. Every individual on the board went through rigorous rounds of assessment to prove their worth. After which they invested a large part of their time researching and compiling the most relevant data for our readers. Conferences and sessions were held from time to time between the editorial board and the contributing authors to present the data in the most comprehensible form. The editorial team has worked tirelessly to provide valuable and valid information to help people across the globe.

Every chapter published in this book has been scrutinized by our experts. Their significance has been extensively debated. The topics covered herein carry significant findings which will fuel the growth of the discipline. They may even be implemented as practical applications or may be referred to as a beginning point for another development. Chapters in this book were first published by InTech; hereby published with permission under the Creative Commons Attribution License or equivalent.

The editorial board has been involved in producing this book since its inception. They have spent rigorous hours researching and exploring the diverse topics which have resulted in the successful publishing of this book. They have passed on their knowledge of decades through this book. To expedite this challenging task, the publisher supported the team at every step. A small team of assistant editors was also appointed to further simplify the editing procedure and attain best results for the readers.

Our editorial team has been hand-picked from every corner of the world. Their multi-ethnicity adds dynamic inputs to the discussions which result in innovative outcomes. These outcomes are then further discussed with the researchers and contributors who give their valuable feedback and opinion regarding the same. The feedback is then collaborated with the researches and they are edited in a comprehensive manner to aid the understanding of the subject.

Apart from the editorial board, the designing team has also invested a significant amount of their time in understanding the subject and creating the most relevant covers. They scrutinized every image to scout for the most suitable representation of the subject and create an appropriate cover for the book.

The publishing team has been involved in this book since its early stages. They were actively engaged in every process, be it collecting the data, connecting with the contributors or procuring relevant information. The team has been an ardent support to the editorial, designing and production team. Their endless efforts to recruit the best for this project, has resulted in the accomplishment of this book. They are a veteran in the field of academics and their pool of knowledge is as vast as their experience in printing. Their expertise and guidance has proved useful at every step. Their uncompromising quality standards have made this book an exceptional effort. Their encouragement from time to time has been an inspiration for everyone.

The publisher and the editorial board hope that this book will prove to be a valuable piece of knowledge for researchers, students, practitioners and scholars across the globe.

List of Contributors

Rúnar Unnþórsson
University of Iceland, School of Engineering and Natural Sciences, Iceland

Zahari Taha
Faculty of Mechanical Engineering, University Malaysia Pahang, Malaysia

Indro Pranoto
Department of Mechanical and Industrial Engineering, Gadjah Mada University, Indonesia

Hyun-Do Yun
Chung-Nam National University, Korea

Wonchang Choi
NC A&T State University, USA

Stefan Jan Kowalski, Jacek Banaszak and Kinga Rajewska
Poznań University of Technology, Institute of Technology and Chemical Engineering, Department of Process Engineering, Poznań, Poland

Giovanni P. Gregori
S.M.E. (Security, Materials, Environment) s.r.l., Roma, Italy
IEVPC – International Earthquake and Volcano Prediction Center, USA
IDASC(CNR), Roma, Italy

Giuliano Ventrice
S.M.E. (Security, Materials, Environment) s.r.l., Roma, Italy
PME Engineering (Progettazione Macchine Elettroniche), Italy
SAE-Technology (System Acoustic Emission Technology), Italy

Sebastiano Pinori
S.M.E. (Security, Materials, Environment) s.r.l., Roma, Italy
"Più s.r.l. costruire il futuro"- Gruppo Alessandrini, Italy

Genesio Alessandrini
S.M.E. (Security, Materials, Environment) s.r.l., Roma, Italy
"Più s.r.l. costruire il futuro"- Gruppo Alessandrini, Italy

Francesco Bianchi
S.M.E. (Security, Materials, Environment) s.r.l., Roma, Italy
Faculty of Architecture, Third University of Rome, Italy

Wojciech Sikorski and Krzysztof Walczak
Poznan University of Technology, Poland

Franciszek Witos
Department of Optoelectronics, Silesian University of Technology, Gliwice, Poland

Zbigniew Gacek
Institute of Power Systems & Control, Silesian University of Technology, Gliwice, Poland

Artur Zdunek
Institute of Agrophysics, Polish Academy of Sciences, Lublin, Poland

Giovanna Zimatore and Maria Patrizia Orlando
CNR-IDASC – Institute of Acoustics and Sensor "Orso Mario Corbino", Rome, Italy

Domenico Stanzial
CNR-IDASC - Institute of Acoustics and Sensor "Orso Mario Corbino", c/o Physics Department University of Ferrara, Italy